Sensory Systems of Primates

ADVANCES IN PRIMATOLOGY

THE PRIMATE BRAIN
Edited by Charles R. Noback and William Montagna

MOLECULAR ANTHROPOLOGY: Genes and Proteins
in the Evolutionary Ascent of the Primates
Edited by Morris Goodman and Richard E. Tashian

SENSORY SYSTEMS OF PRIMATES
Edited by Charles R. Noback

Sensory Systems of Primates

Edited by

Charles R. Noback

Department of Anatomy
Columbia University
New York, New York

PLENUM PRESS • NEW YORK AND LONDON

Library of Congress Cataloging in Publication Data

Main entry under title:

Sensory systems of primates.

(Advances in primatology)
Includes bibliographies and index.
1. Nervous system—Mammals. 2. Primates. I. Noback, Charles Robert, 1916-
III. Series.
QL737.P9P6727   599'.8'04188   78-15383
ISBN 0-306-31127-5

© 1978 Plenum Press, New York
A Division of Plenum Publishing Corporation
227 West 17th Street, New York, N.Y. 10011

Printed in the United States of America

Contributors

JOHN R. COTTER, Department of Anatomical Sciences, State University of New York, Buffalo, New York

LEONARD M. EISENMAN, Department of Anatomy, Thomas Jefferson University, Philadelphia, Pennsylvania

GISELA EPPLE, Monell Chemical Senses Center, University of Pennsylvania, Philadelphia, Pennsylvania

JOHN K. HARTING, Department of Anatomy, University of Wisconsin, Madison, Wisconsin

RALPH L. HOLLOWAY, Department of Anthropology, Columbia University, New York, New York

JON H. KAAS, Department of Psychology, Vanderbilt University, Nashville, Tennessee

SHYAM M. KHANNA, Department of Otolaryngology, College of Physicians and Surgeons, Columbia University, New York, New York

DAVID MOULTON, Monell Chemical Senses Center, University of Pennsylvania, Philadelphia, Pennsylvania

ROBERTA PIERSON PENTNEY, Department of Anatomical Sciences, State University of New York, Buffalo, New York

NORMAN L. STROMINGER, Department of Anatomy, Albany Medical College of Union University, Albany, New York

JUERGEN TONNDORF, Department of Otolaryngology, College of Physicians and Surgeons, Columbia University, New York, New York

JOSEPH T. WEBER, Department of Anatomy, University of Wisconsin, Madison, Wisconsin

Preface

Primates are avid explorers that utilize a variety of sensory clues from the environment. The special senses of olfaction, audition, and particularly vision are thus of paramount significance in the evolution and adaptive radiation of the primates. It was with this in mind that this volume was planned to present some recent research advances.

The chapter on olfactory communication among primates affords new insights concerning a sense which, though primatologists have generally relegated it to a minor role, is of considerable significance in the primates. The chapters on the auditory system are organized to stress three aspects: the receptive organ, the neural pathways, and the role of audition in primate communication. The visual system, the dominant special sense of primates, is analyzed with respect to two regions of the brain, namely, the organization of the superior colliculus and the visual cortex. Finally, the chapter on endocasts in the study of primate brain evolution will alert neurobiologists to the relevant information that can be unearthed from fossils embedded in the terrane.

I wish to thank the publishers, and especially Miss Phyllis Straw and Mr. Seymour Weingarten, for their support, patience, guidance, and professional assistance.

Charles R. Noback

Contents

4.   Vocal Communication in Primates   93

Leonard M. Eisenman

1

Structural Organization and Communicatory Functions of Olfaction in Nonhuman Primates

GISELA EPPLE AND DAVID MOULTON

I. Introduction

Our knowledge of primate chemical communication lags far behind that of visual and vocal patterns. This is not surprising, considering the limitations placed on the human observer by his own sensory capacities. Because of his relatively poorly developed sense of smell, the human observer is much more likely to record a visual or vocal pattern of communication than an odor. Therefore, much of the chemical communication possibly going on in a primate group escapes notice during direct observation. In spite of these limitations, evidence for the use of chemical signals in primate communication has accumulated during recent years.

GISELA EPPLE AND DAVID MOULTON • Monell Chemical Senses Center, University of Pennsylvania, Philadelphia, Pennsylvania 19104.

Among the prosimians and South American monkeys the vomero-nasal and olfactory systems are relatively well developed. However, there is a tendency for their degree of development to decrease, relative to other cortical structures, as a function of the increasing volume of the cortex. From this, one might predict that, while chemical signals from conspecifics and environmental odors should be meaningful in the life of many species, there are certain groups in which they are likely to be highly significant. Although it is not feasible as yet to correlate the morphological findings with a sizeable quantity of behavioral data, many observations suggest that intraspecies chemical communication is highly important to some prosimians and South American monkeys while playing a less powerful role in Old World monkeys and apes.

Specialized odor-producing scent glands are present in most prosimians and South American monkeys but also in a small number of Old World species. The papers on the occurrence and structure of primate skin glands are too numerous to be listed here. More complete reference lists are given by Ellis and Montagna, 1964; Epple, 1974a,c, 1976; Hill, 1954; Montagna, 1972; and Schaffer, 1940.

Most species that possess scent glands also show scent-marking behavior, resulting in the application of glandular secretions to the own body, that of conspecifics, and to items in the environment. Feces, urine, saliva, or discharge from the genital tract may be mixed with skin gland secretions or with each other during marking or, in some species, are used by themselves. For detailed references see Epple (1972, 1974a,c, 1976). Moreover, investigation of conspecifics and of their scent marks by sniffing, mouthing, licking, and ingestion is very frequent during sexual as well as in other social situations in prosimians and New and Old World primates (cf. Epple, 1974a, 1975; Klein, 1971; Klein and Klein, 1971; Blurton-Jones and Trollope, 1968; Michael, 1969; Rahaman and Parthasarathy, 1971; Marler, 1965).

Supposedly, nasal olfaction is the major sense involved in the perception of these chemical signals. Perception via the vomeronasal organ and/or taste, however, cannot be ruled out. As discussed in detail below, a functioning vomeronasal organ and distinctly formed accessory bulbs are present in many prosimians and South American monkeys, and the possibility exists that the system mediates functions distinct from those of the main olfactory system. In fact, Estes (1972) has recently speculated that the vomeronasal organ of mammals might be specifically involved in the perception of signals which are of significance in intraspecies communication.

Some primates, when investigating socially and/or sexually meaningful chemicals, show a behavior which is reminiscent of the rhythmic tongue protrusions of lizards and snakes when smelling. This behavior might possibly bring chemical stimuli into the mouth and to the canales incisivi, from where they could reach the vomeronasal organ. *Nycticebus coucang* (the slow loris), for instance, sniffs the urine of conspecifics while showing rapid oscillating protrusions of the tongue (Seitz, 1969). Several species of South American marmoset monkeys frequently sniff urine, scent marks, or the bodies of conspecifics while showing rhythmical protrusion of the tongue, whose tip may touch the stimulus. *Saimiri sciureus* males show an almost identical behavior when sniffing the urine and the genitals of females (Epple, unpublished). In marmosets the sniffing behavior is occasionally followed by a facial expression very reminiscent of the "Flehem" face which is supposedly involved in perception of mainly sexual stimuli via the vomeronasal organ (Knappe, 1964). *Lemur catta* shows a similar facial expression during the investigation of conspecific chemical stimuli (Jolly, 1966).

Some species not only sniff and lick the various chemical stimuli provided by conspecifics but also ingest excretions and secretions. This suggests that taste might play a role in their perception and/or that some of the stimuli affect the receiving organism via ingestion. *Ateles* males, for instance, frequently taste and drink the urine of females in all stages of the reproductive cycle (Klein, 1971).

The observations outlined above demonstrate that, on the basis of presently available data, an attempt to synthesize anatomical and behavioral findings appears premature. Therefore these two areas are represented here separately with the hope that the facts brought together in this review will stimulate future research and provide some background for its planning.

II. Structural Organization

The degree of development of olfactory structures in primates tends to be inversely proportional to the degree of neocorticalization, of hand mobility, and of frontality of orbits. On the other hand these tendencies are not interdependent.

A. The Nasal Cavity and the Extent of Olfactory Surface

The nasal cavity of primates, as in all mammals, consists of three portions: an anterior chamber, lined by stratified squamous epithelium; a middle chamber, lined by respiratory epithelium; and a posterior chamber, lined with olfactory epithelium. A portion of this last epithelium covers part of the ethmoturbinals which project into the posterior chamber, while a further portion covers the posterior half of the nasal septum. When developed, the vomeronasal organ lies, bilaterally, at the base of the nasal septum (Loo and Kanagasuntheram, 1971; Jordan, 1972).

There is a marked reduction in this area of the olfactory epithelium on passing from prosimian to simian primates. Thus, in the tree shrew (*Tupaia glis*) the olfactory epithelium covers not only the entire ethmoturbinal system but also lines the olfactory recesses. Although some reduction of the ethmoturbinal system is already apparent in the slow loris (*N. coucang*) the olfactory epithelium is still relatively extensive. In the macaque and gibbon, however, the ethmoturbinal system is much simplified, and the olfactory epithelium does not extend into the olfactory recesses. Paralleling this deemphasis of olfactory structures, the vomeronasal organ is reduced to a cartilaginous vestige in the macaque and reported absent (but presumably vestigial) in the gibbon (Meinel and Woehrmann-Repenning, 1973). In contrast, it is well developed in *Nycticebus coucang, Nycticebus tardigradus, Tupaia glis,* and *Cebus capucinus* (Jordan, 1972; Loo, 1974).

If the direction of an odor source can be identified by slight differences in the time of arrival of odorous molecules at the two nares, as has been claimed for man, the degree of separation of these nares may be significant. In this context, the majority of Cebidae, which show the platyrrhine condition (nostrils wide apart), may have an advantage over the Cercopithecidae and apes, which show the catarrhine condition (nostrils separated by only a narrow septum).

B. Olfactory Epithelium

The olfactory epithelium varies widely in thickness, being 30–110 μm in the tree shrew (Meinel and Woehrmann-Repenning, 1973).

The basic organization of this epithelium in primates adheres to the general vertebrate pattern of three cell types—receptor, supporting, and basal—overlain by a mucus sheet. This sheet is probably at least 20–50 μm thick in *Macaca mulatta* (Reese and Brightman, 1970) and is derived, in part, from specialized multicellular glands (Bowman's glands) in the lamina propria. In this species, the mucus is PAS (*p*-aminosalycylic acid) positive, indicating the presence of a complex mucopolysaccharide or glycoprotein. It also contains oxidative and some hydrolytic enzymes (Shantha and Nakajima, 1970).

Each receptor is a bipolar neuron whose dendrite terminates in a club-shaped swelling or knob bearing cilia. In the squirrel monkey there are 8–20 cilia per cell each having a minimal length of 50 μm. In *Tupaia* they are 100 μm long (de Lorenzo, 1970; Meinel and Woehrmann-Repenning, 1973). Microvilli may also be present (Shantha and Nakajima, 1970; Reese and Brightman, 1970). The cilia lie in parallel arrays near the cell surface and are thought by many to support sites where the odorant–receptor interaction occurs. If so, the number of such sites must be vast even in a simian. If we assume 10 million olfactory receptors in the squirrel monkey, the total surface area of the cilia can be calculated from published data. This is of the order of 7.3×10^{11} μm^2 (7.3×0.1m^2), or an area greater than the animal's entire body surface.

There is an unconfirmed report that the rhesus monkey, in common with certain other species, has a second type of olfactory receptor which is flask- instead of rod-shaped (Vinnikov, 1956). In addition, Shantha and Nakajima (1970) found that while the majority of receptors were moderately positive for oxidation enzyme activity in this species, some were strongly positive. What functional significance such differences have, if any, is not clear.

Receptors are separated from one another by supporting cells to which they are related by tight junctions. Supporting cells bear microvilli which are 10 μm long in the rhesus monkey (Reese and Brightman, 1970). Although some mitotic activity has been seen in supporting cells of tree shrews (*T. glis*) it is mainly concentrated in their basal cells (Meinel and Woehrmann-Repenning, 1973). Presumably products of basal cell division migrate peripherally and replace dying receptor cells to provide a continuous turnover, as occurs in the mouse (see Moulton, 1974). Following destruction of the olfactory mucosa by zinc sulfate necrosis, receptor cells in the rhesus monkey regenerated to an apparently normal state in 6 months to 1 year (Schultz, 1960).

The olfactory system appears to have a unique relation with the blood–brain barrier insofar as dyes placed on the olfactory epithelium reach the brain rather rapidly. Polio viruses placed intranasally in monkeys traveled in the axoplasm of the primary neurons and were recovered from the olfactory bulb (Bodian and Howe, 1941a,b). More recently de Lorenzo (1970) investigated the rate and mechanism of transfer by placing colloidal gold particles intranasally in the squirrel monkey. They were incorporated into the cytoplasm of the receptor cell, apparently by pinocytosis, and within an hour appeared in the glomeruli of the olfactory bulb, where they accumulated preferentially in the mitochondria of the mitral cell dendrites. The transport rate was about 2.5mm/h, which is comparable to that of the polio virus (2.4 mm/h) in the sciatic nerve (Bodian and Howe, 1941a).

There has been no study made of the electrical activity of the olfactory epithelium of any prosimian or simian species but presumably it does not differ significantly from that of other vertebrates (see Moulton and Tucker, 1964).

C. Vomeronasal (Jacobson's) Organ and Epithelium, and the Accessory Olfactory Bulb

The bilateral vomeronasal organ projects to the accessory olfactory bulb and is usually considered as an accessory olfactory organ. Although its role in mammals is not well understood, it may mediate functions distinct from those of the olfactory bulb. This possibility is supported by the fact that the main and accessory bulbs are independent on one another in size throughout the range of primate species (Stephan, 1965). The organ lies partially enclosed in a cartilaginous capsule at the base of the septum in the hard palate, medial to the incisive ducts. In primates it usually connects, by way of the vomeronasal duct, with the incisive duct, which in turn communicates with the oral and nasal cavities. Thus it may respond both to food odors in the mouth and to odors in the nasal cavity.

The sensory epithelium of the vomeronasal organ in *Tupaia belangeri* is similar to that of other vertebrate species so far studied and to that of the olfactory epithelium. However, the vomeronasal receptor cells lack cilia, although they contain centrioles and precursor bodies of cilia. The supporting cells apparently show a rather low to moderate secretory activity as compared with supporting cells in the olfactory epithelium (Kolnberger, 1971; Kolnberger and Altner, 1971). The density of the vomeronasal receptors is lower in *Tupaia* (25,000 receptors/mm²; Kolnberger, 1971) than in the lemur *Microcebus murinus* (90,000 receptors/mm² or 209,000 per organ; Schilling, 1970).

Stephan (1965) found a distinctly formed accessory bulb in 12 species of prosimians (well developed except in *Tarsius*) as well as in all the platyrrhine monkeys that he examined, but in the catarrhini it was absent.

D. Olfactory Bulb

Estimates of the volumes of a range of brain structures in 41 different species of primates allowed Stephan and Andy (1969) to compile "progression indices." Each value provides a direct numerical estimate of how many times larger a given brain structure of a certain species is than the corresponding structure in a typical basal insectivore of the same body weight. Of all the structures measured in this way the only one showing any clear-cut regression was the olfactory bulb. It has a progression index corresponding to an average reduction of ⅓ in the prosimians and ⁹⁄₁₀ in the simians. In striking contrast, the corresponding figures for the neocortex is 14½ times as large as basal insectivores for prosimians and 45½ times as large for simians (Fig. 1).

While progressive neocorticalization and progressive reduction in bulb size are clearly related, they are not necessarily interdependent. (The aye aye and dwarf galago, for example, provide exceptions.)

The distribution of enzymes in the olfactory bulb of the squirrel monkey has been studied by Shantha Veerappa and Bourne (1965) and Iijima *et al.* (1967). The various layers show different degrees of enzyme activity indicating functional and metabolic differences. A pacinian corpuscle has also been noted on the olfactory bulb of this species (Shantha Veerappa and Bourne, 1966).

Although a few scattered observations exist (e.g., Vaccarezza and Saavedra, 1968), there appears to have been no comprehensive study made of bulbar structure in any simian or prosimian species, but it is unlikely to depart significantly from the general mammalian plan (see Shepherd, 1972).

The slow oscillatory responses recorded from the olfactory bulb of

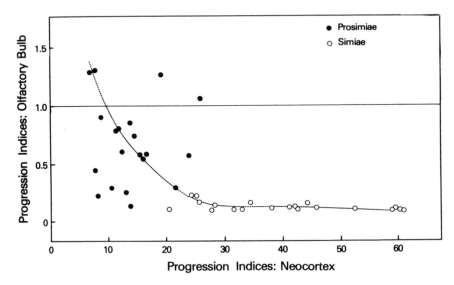

Fig. 1.   Relation between progression indices for olfactory bulb and neocortex in prosimians and simians. (Data from Stephan and Andy, 1969.)

alert rhesus monkeys show a background activity of low-amplitude, asynchronous discharges. While odors with low molecular weight and sharp penetrating odors inhibited this activity, others increased it, eliciting frequences in the range of 20–55 Hz. The claim (Hughes and Mazurowski, 1962), that different odors elicited different peak frequencies—some characteristic of the stimulus—has yet to be confirmed.

Recordings of single units in the bulb of both anesthetized and restrained but unanesthetized macaques show only 60% of 67 cells responding to one or more of eight odors tested. Of these cells, 12.5% responded to one odor and one cell responded to all odors. The dominant response was excitation (Tanabe et al., 1975a). In other words, the majority of second-order bulbar neurons show a relatively low degree of odor specificity.

E. Secondary and Higher Projections of the Olfactory Bulb

Secondary olfactory projections in primates have been investigated by modern methods for degenerating axons (e.g., Fink–Heimer) only in the case of the galago and the tree shrew (Ferrer, 1969). Unfortunately this study did not distinguish between the projections of the main and accessory bulbs, which have been shown to be distinct in other species. In general, however, the findings agree with other recent work on mammals in showing projections to the olfactory tubercle, the prepyriform lobes, the anterior olfactory nucleus, the nucleus of the lateral olfactory tract, and the corticomedial segment of the amygdaloid complex. In other species, specific projections of the main bulb have also been found to the rostroventral end of the anterior hippocampus (tenia tecta), the dorsomedial and lateral entorhinal area, the transition area between the prepyriform cortex and the horizontal limb of the diagonal band, and the anterior and posterolateral cortical amygdaloid nuclei (see Moulton, 1978). While certain of these projections have only recently been described in any mammalian species and therefore might also occur in primates, Heimer (1969) has pointed out that there may be important interspecific differences in the distribution of the olfactory bulb fibers among mammals. In particular, he found that the major part of the olfactory tubercle in the rhesus monkey lies outside the reach of olfactory bulb fibers, contrary to the situation in rat and rabbit.

Since there appear to be many parallel projection pathways to higher olfactory centers, ablation studies yielding negative results may be of limited significance: for example, the finding that bilateral amygdalectomy does not influence olfactory discrimination in monkeys (Schuckman et al., 1969).

Recent studies on rabbit, opossum, and rat have shown that the projections of the accessory bulb are quite distinct from those of the main bulb. They terminate in the bed nucleus of the accessory olfactory tract, the bed nucleus of the stria terminalis, the medial amygdaloid nucleus, and the posteromedial part of the cortical amygdaloid nucleus (see Moulton, 1978). Heimer (1969), however, could find no evidence for a projection to the bed nucleus of the stria terminalis or to the central amygdaloid nuclei in the rhesus monkey.

From these primary olfactory projection sites, further connections channel olfactory information to various diencephalic and mesencephalic structures where this information may influence the wide range of behaviors with which these structures are associated. For example, stimulation of the olfactory bulb in the squirrel monkey and macaque evoked responses in the mediodorsal nucleus of the thalamus with latencies as short as 4 msec. It is known that, in the rat, there is a direct projection to this nucleus from the pyriform cortex (Benjamin and

Jackson, 1974; Tanabe *et al.*, 1975b). An olfactory projection area has also been identified in the orbitofrontal cortex of the macaque. However, the pathway from the bulb appears to pass through the anterior pyriform cortex (and possibly the medial portion of the amygdala) and hypothalamus, and not through the thalamus.

III. Communicatory Functions of Olfactory Signals

While anatomical findings and behavioral observations strongly imply the importance of odors in the life of many primates, experimental work on intraspecies chemical communication has only started very recently. It appears that primates, like other mammalian species (cf. Bronson, 1971; Eisenberg and Kleiman, 1972; Müller-Schwarze, 1974; Mykytowycz, 1970), make extensive use of chemical signals to communicate details about the individual who produced them. These signals carry information such as species identity, sex, age, individual identity, reproductive condition, social status, and emotional state. They are well suited to be used in a variety of behavioral contexts. In combination with other communicants such as calls or visual displays, and according to the behavioral situation and physiological condition in which sender and recipient find themselves, a signal can fulfill different functions. For instance, chemical information on the sex of an individual might attract an animal of the opposite sex in the "correct" reproductive condition but repel an animal of the same sex or even elicit aggression. Individual odors may serve as social or sexual attractants among animals who have established friendly relationships with each other, while they may be regarded as threat signals among individuals who have interacted agonistically. Thus, the function of a chemical signal is largely determined by its behavioral context and by the physiological condition and previous experiences of the recipient.

Because of this, any one chemical signal may be involved in a variety of behaviors such as group cohesion, spacing and territoriality, intergroup and intragroup aggression, parent–infant interactions, recognition of and attraction to a sexual partner in the right stage of reproductive activity, sexual arousal, temporary or permanent male–female pair bonding, and reproductive synchronization.

There is circumstantial evidence for the involvement of chemical signals in all of these behaviors in a number of species. Much of the material, facts as well as speculations, has recently been reviewed in some detail, and the various aspects of primate behavior and reproduction in which external chemical messengers seem to be of importance have been discussed (Epple, 1974a,b,c, 1976). Therefore, the present review shall not deal with implied functions but concentrate on experimental work in primate chemical communication.

A. Species Identity

Experimental studies have shown that the slow loris, *Nycticebus coucang* (Seitz, 1969), and the greater galago, *Galago crassicaudatus crassicaudatus* and *Galago crassicaudatus argentatus* (Clark, 1974), show spontaneous discriminative responses when presented with odors of conspecifics and closely related species or subspecies (urine samples and scent marks), demonstrating recognition of the differences between them. *Lemur fulvus*, on the other hand, does not seem to discriminate between the odors of different subspecies, suggesting that they may be similar (Harrington, 1974).

B. Sexual Identity

Identification of maleness and femaleness by odors may be widespread among primates. Males of the tree shrews, *T. belangeri*, for instance, discriminated between the secretions of the sternal gland and urine from mature, immature, and castrated males and from females (Stralendorff, cf. von Holst, 1974).* Male and female slow loris (*N. coucang*), when presented with samples of their own urine, urine from a strange male, and urine from a strange female, discriminated between them, sniffing the male urine longer than female urine or their own (Seitz, 1969).

Clark (1974) gave male and female galagos (*G. crassicaudatus argentatus*) a choice between two plastic perches—one of them carrying scent marks of males, the second carrying female marks. The marks were complex mixtures resulting from various types of scent-marking behavior in whatever combination the donor animals choose. (The

---

* *Tupaia* is included here for the purpose of completeness. By doing so, the authors do not wish to express an opinion about the taxonomic proximity of the Tupaidae to Primates. This controversy has been extensively discussed by several authors and has been reviewed by Martin (1968).

species shows five different types using urine as well as skin glands.) The galagos discriminated between these complex stimuli, spending more time sniffing female odors and showing a higher frequency of licking, urine marking, anogenital rubbing, and chest rubbing on the female-scented perch.

Harrington (1974) presented male *L. fulvus* with gauze pads which had been left in the cage of a conspecific overnight. The males sniffed pads carrying male odor more frequently than pads with female odor when the pads were presented to them successively. One male, when presented simultaneously with a male-scented pad and female-scented pad, preferred male odor. The source of the sexual identifiers remained undetermined since the gauze pads probably carried a mixture of urine, feces, and various skin gland secretions.

Epple (1971, 1973, 1974a,b,c) studied the communicatory messages in the complex scent marks of the saddle-backed tamarin (*Saguinus fuscicollis*). The marks of males and females consist of mixtures of secretions from scent glands in the circumgenital, suprapubic, and sternal areas, urine, and (in the female) vaginal discharge.

Discrimination between male and female odors was tested in a series of experiments during which the marmosets received a choice between two perches of identical dimensions, one carrying adult male scent marks and the other adult female scent marks. Under various conditions of testing, male and female subjects scent-marked significantly more frequently on the perch carrying male odor. This response was shown when each stimulus perch had been marked by only one strange donor monkey (Epple, 1974b). The same result was obtained when each stimulus perch carried the marks of two donors, and also when the male perch had been marked by one male but the female perch by two females and vice versa (Epple, 1971). When each perch carried a sample of marks from 8 males pooled in an organic solvent and an equivalent sample from 8 females, the male sample was scent-marked preferentially (Epple, 1974b). Females, but not males, also scent-marked preferentially on top of male urine when a choice between male and female urine was presented in the absence of intact scent marks (Epple, 1978a).

These results suggest the presence of sexual identifiers in the scent marks and in the urine of tamarins and indicate that sexual identification is based on qualitative differences rather than quantitative ones. The urinary messages possibly stem from contamination with scent gland secretions during elimination. Future experiments are needed to establish the exact source of the information.

C. Identification of Reproductive Condition

Some primates not only communicate maleness and femaleness by odors, but also the reproductive condition of an individual. Evidence so far is limited to females, but it is conceivable that males also signal their ability and readiness to mate, especially in species who are seasonally spermatogenic, such as the squirrel monkey (Baldwin, 1970).

In the great majority of species no experimental work has been done. However, many field and laboratory observations on prosimians, South American monkeys, and Old World primates suggest the production of "sex attractants" signaling the receptive phase of the ovulatory cycle of females and simultaneously arousing male sexual activity: an increase in male and/or female scent-marking behavior, sniffing and mouthing of female genitalia by males, and even ingestion or tasting of female urine or vaginal discharge is part of the sexual behavior of many species. In some of them, sniffing is mutual, with females being little less active than males. (For detailed references see Epple, 1974a,c, 1976.)

In addition, observations on spider monkeys and on several species of marmosets imply that odors may also communicate other phases of the reproductive cycle, such as pregnancy (cf. Epple, 1974c, 1976; Klein, 1971).

To date, the rhesus monkey (*M. mulatta*) is the only species in which "sex attractants" have been studied experimentally. The work of Michael and his co-workers (see below) has suggested that sexual attractiveness in the female and sexual arousal in the male depend strongly on chemical signals of vaginal origin.

In one experiment, Michael and Keverne (1968) trained two males to press a lever to obtain access to females. The males worked consistently to interact with one overiectomized female who had been rendered sexually attractive by injection of extrogen. They did not press consistently for two ovariectomized females who did not receive estrogen. This preference was essentially unchanged when the males were made temporarily anosmic, possibly because the males remembered the estrogenized female to be attractive. When both anhormonal females were given estrogen intravaginally, which should have made them sexually attrative to the males (Michael and Saayman, 1968), the males did not respond to this change in female attractiveness. These results suggest that anosmia, although it does not impair sexual motivation, impairs the male's ability to discriminate attractive from unattractive females. However, after reversal of anosmia, both males gained access to the females receiving intravaginal estrogen, apparently being capable now to perceive their attractiveness.

In another experiment (Michael and Keverne, 1970), two other males lever-pressed consistently for ovariectomized females only after vaginal lavages from estrogen-treated females were applied to the sexual skin of these females. Sexual interactions commenced after this treatment, suggesting that the vaginal lavages contained sexually attracting and arousing substances. Ether extracts of such lavages also led to an increase in sexual behavior as compared to control treatment of the females with ether when three males were given free access to three ovariectomized females (Keverne and Michael, 1971).

Curtis et al. (1971) proposed that the active constituents of the vaginal lavages are a mixture of five aliphatic acids and stated that a synthetic mixture of these acids mimicked the behavioral effects of the natural attractants.

Goldfoot et al. (1976) recently reported that they were unable to replicate the findings of Michael and his co-workers. They tested the sexual behavior of 19 males and 27 females during sexual encounters under various conditions. Either vaginal lavage from an ovariectomized, estrogenized donor female or water was applied to the sexual skin of the ovariectomized subject females. The lavages did not induce a significant increase in the sexual interactions of the pairs as compared to water under any of the conditions tested by Goldfoot et al. (1976). Vaginal lavages contaminated by ejaculate from previous copulations were somewhat but not dramatically more active. A synthetic mixture of aliphatic acids, either prepared according to Curtis et al. (1971) or containing the acids in much higher concentration, failed to stimulate copulation to ejaculation. These results suggest that for the majority of males, female attractiveness is little affected by the presence or absence of vaginal aliphatic acids. Moreover, in cycling females an increase in the concentration of these acids seems to be associated with the luteal phase of the cycle rather than with the time of ovulation (Goldfoot et al., 1976). This argues against the assumption that they signal the most favorable time for conception.

Goldfoot *et al.* (1976) have discussed in detail some of the possible reasons for discrepancies between their findings and those of Michael and co-workers. Several methodological differences between the two studies are pointed out. Among them is the fact that Michael and co-workers had much fewer animals at their disposal than Goldfoot *et al.* Moreover, the males had encountered the recipient females repeatedly throughout several experiments, probably establishing long-lasting personal relationships with them. Therefore, the effects of learning in these experiments are hard to assess. Goldfoot *et al.* (1976) suggest the possibility that experience with a female prior to the application of vaginal lavages could have extinguished the male's interest in her and that vaginal material might thereafter have served as a disinhibitory stimulus.

Furthermore, one wonders whether as yet unidentified components of vaginal discharge might not be responsible for the behavioral effects. Keverne (1974) reports that phenylpropanoic acid and parahydroxy-phenylpropanoic acid are present in natural vaginal secretions. These compounds were not stimuli by themselves, but their addition to the synthetic aliphatic acid mixture improved its effectiveness relative to the synthetic mixture alone. Considering all these points, it seems possible that the mixture of aliphatic acids alone is capable of stimulating sexual activities in a limited number of males under very specific conditions and strongly influenced by sexual experience with a female, while other individuals require additional chemical and/or behavioral signals as stimuli.

D. Individual Identity

A number of species produce odors which identify the individual. A male slow loris (*N. cougang*), for instance, could discriminate between samples of his own urine and that of another male, spending more time sniffing the strange male's urine when presented with successive samples (Seitz, 1969). Harrington (1974) demonstrated the presence of individual chemical identifiers in *L. fulvus*. He presented the lemurs with a succession of gauze pads carrying the odor of one individual. After habituation to this individual's odor was evident by a decrease in the response to the stimuli, pads carrying another individual's odor were presented. Sniffing differences between prehabituation and posthabituation trials showed that the lemurs could discriminate between the odors of individual females as well as between individual male odors. Using this habituation technique, Mertl (1975) showed that material collected from the antebrachial scent glands of male *L. catta* is individually specific. The stimulus material contained old and fresh secretions from the antebrachial organ and probably secretions from the brachial gland, which are often actively mixed with those of the antebrachial organ (Mertl, 1975). Clark (1974), also using the habituation technique, demonstrated the existence of individual identifiers in the complex scent marks of male and female *G. crassicaudatus* and in the chest gland secretions of females. Doyle (1974) states that bush babies (*Galago senegalensis*) recognize each other by odors. Epple (1973) showed that the tamarin, *S. fuscicollis*, can discriminate between the scent marks of two individuals of the same sex, offered simultaneously in a two-choice test. To motivate the marmosets to show a discriminative response, use was made of their tendency to strongly aggress against adult conspecifics who are not members of their social group. The monkeys were given a series of aggressive encounters with either a male or a female belonging to another group. Following each encounter, they were offered the choice between a perch marked by the recent opponent and one marked by a familiar donor of the same sex who was not a group member either. When they were tested one hour after termination of the encounter, as well as when tested several days after an encounter, the marmosets spent more time in investigating, sniffing, and scent-marking perches carrying the odor of their opponent. This preference for the opponent's scent marks, shown even days after an encounter, indicates that discrimination was based on individual odor differences rather than on stress-specific changes in the opponent. It also shows that the subjects could remember the odor of individual conspecifics for several days (Epple, 1973).

The work of Kaplan and Russell (1974) demonstrated individual differences in the odors of squirrel monkeys (*S. sciureus*) and suggests a possible role of individual body odors in filial attachment of infants. Infants reared on surrogate mothers covered with artificial fur seemed to become attached to, and comforted by, the complex odors of the fur covers. In a preference test they preferred covers on which they had lived for several days over clean ones of the same color, supposedly being comforted by the familiar smell. Furthermore, they distinguished between covers soiled by themselves and covers soiled by other infants, preferring the former (Kaplan and Russell, 1974).

E. Identification of Emotional and Social Condition

Although experimental evidence is scant there is some indication that changes in emotional condition are reflected in changes of the quality and/or quantity of body odors. Manley's (1974) observations on the potto (*Perodicticus potto*) and the angwantibo (*Arctocebus calabarensis*), for instance, suggest that the genital scent glands of these prosimians produce fear and stress odors.

Very little experimental work is available on the communication of social status by chemical signals. However, many species of primates apparently scent-mark with increasing frequency when they are both aggressive and dominant (for detailed references, see Epple, 1974a,c). This suggests that scent-marking behavior per se and/or the quantity or quality of chemicals deposited thereby play a role in communicating aggressive motivation and, maybe, the social status of the marking animal. Work done in our own laboratory supports this idea (Epple, 1970, 1973, 1978b). We found that in groups of common marmosets (*Callithrix jacchus jacchus*) containing several nonrelated adults, the dominant male and the dominant female scent-mark much more frequently than submissive group members. Moreover, when a strange conspecific was introduced into these groups for a 10-min social encounter, it was mainly the α-male who aggressed severely against male intruders while mainly the α-female aggressed against female intruders. The scent-marking frequencies of the dominant males and females were dramatically increased during the hour following a 10-min encounter as compared to trial-free situations, but marking was almost completely suppressed in the submissive intruders (Epple, 1970).

In another experiment we introduced a strange conspecific to permanently mated pairs of *S. fuscicollis* for a series of social encounters. During the encounters both partners aggressed against the stranger, and their scent-marking frequency was dramatically increased as compared to trial-free conditions (Epple, 1978b). Moreover, *S. fuscicollis* is able to discriminate the odors of unknown males of different social rank, either on the basis of odor quality or on the basis of odor quantity. When we offered the tamarins a choice between two perches, one carrying the scent marks of an unfamiliar dominant male and the second carrying the scent marks of an unfamiliar subdominant male, they spent more time sniffing and marking the dominant male's perch.

The results of these studies suggest that one of the functions of scent marking in *S. fuscicollis* and in *C. jacchus jacchus* is the communication of aggressive motivation. The quality and/or the quantity of the odors produced during the aggressive marking, or even the marking behavior itself, might communicate the motivation of the marker to group members and strange conspecifics. By doing so, the odor might serve as a threat display, possibly being a substitute for overt aggression in the establishment and maintenance of social dominance.

It is easy to envision how chemical signals might serve as threat displays in intragroup and intergroup communication: A high frequency of marking, regardless of its motivation, results in a large amount of this particular individual's scent in the environment. The marks identify the individual, its sex, and maybe even its social status, and advertise its presence throughout the living space, even if the animal itself is not present. Marmosets sniff the marks of conspecifics frequently, and therefore social partners must be aware of the amount and identity of the odor. An individual, be it a submissive member of the group or an intruder, who has experienced domination or even defeat by a superior and is exposed to the superior's odor throughout much of its living space, might be quite affected. In this way the scent marks of aggressive, dominant marmosets may function as substitutes for overt aggression, maintaining the hierarchy within the groups and enforcing group integrity.

It is conceivable that similar mechanisms are involved in some of the various other species of primates who also show a strong increase in scent-marking during aggressive interactions (cf. Epple, 1974a,c).

IV. References

Baldwin, J. D. 1970. Reproductive synchronization in squirrel monkeys (*Saimiri*). *Primates 11:* 317–326.

Benjamin, R. M., and Jackson, J. C. 1974. Unit discharges in the mediodorsal nucleus of the squirrel monkey evoked by electrical stimulation of the olfactory bulb. *Brain Res. 75:*181–191.

Blurton-Jones, N. B., and Trollope, J. 1968. Social behaviour of stump-tailed macaques in captivity. *Primates 9:*365–394.

Bodian, D., and Howe, H. A. 1941a. Experimental studies on intraneural spread of poliomyelitis virus. *Bull. Johns Hopkins Hosp. 88*:248–267.

Bodian, D., and Howe, H. A. 1941b. The rate of progression of poliomyelitis virus in nerves. *Bull. Johns Hopkins Hosp. 69*:79–85.

Bronson, F. H. 1971. Rodent pheromones. *Biol. Reprod. 4*:344–357.

Clark, A. 1974. Olfactory communication in *Galago crassicaudatus*. Thesis, University of Chicago.

Curtis, R. F., Ballantine, J. A., Keverne, E. B., Bonsall, R. W., and Michael, R. P. 1971. Identification of primate sexual pheromones and the properties of synthetic attractants. *Nature (London) 232*:396–398.

de Lorenzo, A. J. D. 1970. The olfactory neuron and the blood–brain barrier. *In* G. E. W. Wolstenholme and J. Knight (eds.). *Taste and Smell in Vertebrates.* J. and A. Churchill, London. Pp. 151–176.

Doyle, G. A. 1974. The behavior of the lesser bushbaby (*Galago senegalensis moholi*). *In* R. D. Martin, G. A. Doyle, and A. C. Walker (eds.). *Prosimian Biology.* Gloucester Crescent, Duckworth. Pp. 213–231.

Eisenberg, J. F., and Kleiman, D. G. 1972. Olfactory communication in mammals. *Annu. Rev. Ecol. Sys. 3*:1–32.

Ellis, R. A., and Montagna, W. 1964. The sweat glands of the Lorisidae. *In* J. Buettner-Janusch (ed.). *Evolutionary and Genetic Biology of the Primates,* Vol. II. Academic Press, New York. Pp. 197–228.

Epple, G. 1970. Quantitative studies on scent marking in the marmoset (*Callithrix jacchus*). *Folia Primatol. 13*:48–62.

Epple, G. 1971. Discrimination of the odor of males and females by the marmoset *Saguinus fuscicollis* ssp. *Proc. Int. Congr. Primatol. 3*:166–171.

Epple, G. 1972. Social communication by olfactory signals in marmosets. *Int. Zoo Yearb. 12*:36–42.

Epple, G. 1973. The role of pheromones in the social communication of marmoset monkeys (*Callithricidae*). *J. Reprod. Fertil. Suppl. 19*:447–454.

Epple, G. 1974a. Primate pheromones. *In* M. C. Birch (ed.). *Pheromones.* North-Holland Amsterdam. Pp. 366–385

Epple, G. 1974b. Pheromones in primate reproduction and social behavior. *In* W. Montagna and W. A. Sadler (eds.). *Reproductive Behavior.* Plenum Press, New York. Pp. 131–155.

Epple, G. 1974c. Olfactory communication in South American primates. *Ann. N.Y. Acad. Sci. 237*:261–278.

Epple, G. 1975. The behavior of marmoset monkeys (*Callithricidae*). *In* L. A. Rosenblum (ed.). *Primate Behavior,* Vol. 4. Academic Press, New York. Pp. 195–239.

Epple, G. 1976. Chemical communication and reproductive processes in nonhuman primates. *In* R. L. Doty (ed.). *Mammalian Olfaction, Reproductive Processes and Behavior.* Academic Press, New York. Pp. 257–282.

Epple, G. 1978a. Studies on the nature of chemical signals in scent marks and urine of *Saguinus fuscicollis* (Callithricidae, Primates). *J. Chem. Ecol. 4*:383–394.

Epple, G. 1978b. Notes on the establishment and maintenance of the pair bond in *Saguinus fuscicollis. In* D. Kleiman (ed.). *Biology and Conservation of the Callitrichidae.* Smithsonian Press, Washington, D.C. In press.

Estes, R. D. 1972. The role of the vomeronasal organ in mammalian reproduction. *Mammalia 3:*315–341.

Ferrer, N. G. 1969. Secondary olfactory projections in the galago (*Galago crassicaudatus*) and the tree shrew (*Tupaia glis*). *J. Comp. Neurol. 136:*337–348.

Goldfoot, D. A., Kravets, M. A., Goy, R. W., and Freeman, S. K. 1976. Lack of effect of vaginal lavages and aliphatic acids on ejaculatory responses in rhesus monkeys: Behavioral and chemical analyses. *Horm. Behav. 7:*1–27.

Harrington, J. 1974. Olfactory communication in *Lemur fulvus*. In R. D. Martin, G. A. Doyle, and A. C. Walker (eds.). *Prosimian Biology*. Pp. 331–346. Gloucester Crescent, Duckworth.

Heimer, L. 1969. The secondary olfactory connections in mammals, reptiles, and sharks. *Ann. N.Y. Acad. Sci. 167:*129–146.

Hill, W. C. O. 1954. Sternal glands in the genus *Madrillus*. *J. Anat. 88:*582.

Hughes, R. R., and Mazurowski, J. A. 1962. Studies on the supracallosal mesial cortex of unanesthetized, conscious mammals. II. Monkey. C. Frequency analysis of responses from the olfactory bulb. *Electroencephalogr. Clin. Neurophysiol. 14:*646–653.

Iijima, K., Shantha, T. R., and Bourne, G. H. 1967. Histochemical studies on the distribution of some enzymes of the glycolytic pathways in the olfactory bulb of the squirrel monkey (*Saimiri sciureus*). *Histochemie 10:*224–229.

Jolly, A. 1966. *Lemur Behavior: A Madagascar Field Study*. University of Chicago Press, Chicago.

Jordan, J. 1972. The vomeronasal organ (of Jacobson) in primates. *Folia Morphol. (Warsaw) Engl. Transl. 31:*418–432.

Kaplan, J., and Russell, M. 1974. Olfactory recognition in the infant squirrel monkey. *Dev. Psychobiol. 7:*15–19.

Keverne, E. B. 1974. Sex-attractants in primates. *New Sci. 61:*22–24.

Keverne, E. B., and Michael, R. P. 1971. Sex-attractant properties of ether extracts of vaginal secretions from rhesus monkeys. *J. Endocrinol. 51:*313–322.

Klein, L. L. 1971. Observations on copulation and seasonal reproduction of two species of spider monkeys *Ateles belzebuth* and *A. geoffroyi*. *Folia Primatol. 15:*233–248.

Klein, L. L., and Klein, D. 1971. Aspects of social behavior in a colony of spider monkeys. *Int. Zoo Yearb. 11:*175–181.

Knappe, H. 1964. Zur Funktion des Jacobsonschen Organs (Organon vomeronasale Jacobsoni). *Zool. Gart. 28:*188–194.

Kolnberger, I. 1971. Vergleichende Untersuchungen am Riechepithel. Insbesondere des Jacobsonschen Organs von Amphibien, Reptilien und Säugetieren. *Z. Zellforsch. Mikrosk. Anat. 122:*53–67.

Kolnberger, I., and Altner, H. 1971. Ciliary-structure precursor bodies as stable constituents in the sensory cells of the vomero-nasal organ of reptiles and mammals. *Z. Zellforsch. Mikrosk. Anat. 118:*254–262.

Loo, S. K. 1974. Comparative study of the histology of the nasal fossa in four primates. *Folia Primatol. 21:*290–303.

Loo, S. K., and Kanagasuntheram, R. 1971. The nasal fossa of *Tupaia glis* and *Nycticebus coucang*. *Folia Primatol. 16:*74–84.

Manley, G. H. 1974. Functions of the external genital glands of *Perodicticus* and *Arctocebus*. *In* R. D. Martin, G. A. Doyle, and A. C. Walker (eds.). *Prosimian Biology.* Gloucester Crescent, Duckworth. Pp. 313–329.

Marler, P. 1965. Communication in monkeys and apes. *In* I. DeVore (ed.). *Primate Behavior. Field Studies of Monkeys and Apes.* Holt, Rinehart and Winston, New York. Pp. 544–584.

Martin, R. D. 1968. Reproduction and ontogeny in tree shrews (*Tupaia belangeri*) with reference to their general behaviour and taxonomic relationships. *Z. Tierpsychol.* 25:409–495.

Meinel, W., and Woehrmann-Repenning, A. 1973. Zur Morphologie und Histologie des Geruchorgans von *Tupaia glis* (Dinard 1820). *Folia Primatol.* 20:294–311.

Mertl, A. 1975. Discrimination of individuals by scent in a primate. *Behav. Biol.* 14:505–509.

Michael, R. P. 1969. The role of pheromones in the communication of primate behaviour. *In Recent Advances in Primatology,* Vol. 1. S. Karger, Basel. Pp. 101–107.

Michael, R. P., and Keverne, E. B. 1968. Pheromones in the communication of sexual status in primates. *Nature (London)* 218:746–749

Michael, R. P., and Keverne, E. P. 1970. Primate sex pheromones of vaginal origin. *Nature (London)* 225:84–85.

Michael, R. P., and Saayman, G. S. 1968. Differential effects on behaviour of the subcutaneous and intravaginal administration of oestrogen in the rhesus monkey (*Macaca mulatta*). *J. Endocrinol.* 41:231–246.

Montagna, W. 1972. The skin of nonhuman primates. *Am. Zool.* 12:109–124.

Moulton, D. G. 1974. Dynamics of cell populations in the olfactory epithelium. *Ann. N.Y. Acad. Sci.* 237:52–61.

Moulton, D. G. 1978. Olfaction. *In* B. Masterton (ed.). *Sensory Integration: Handbook of Behavioral Neurobiology 1.* In press.

Moulton, D. G., and Tucker, D. 1964. Electrophysiology of the olfactory system. *Ann. N.Y. Acad. Sci.* 116:380–428.

Müller-Schwarze, D. 1974. Olfactory recognition of species, groups, individuals and physiological states among mammals. *In* M. C. Birch (ed.). *Pheromones.* American Elsevier, New York. Pp. 316–326.

Mykytowycz, R. 1970. The role of skin glands in mammalian communication. *In* J. W. Johnston, D. G. Moulton, and A. Turk (eds.). *Communication by Chemical Signals.* Appleton-Century-Crofts, New York. Pp. 327–360.

Rahaman, H., and Parthasarathy, M. D. 1971. The role of olfactory signals in the mating behavior of bonnet monkeys (*Macaca radiata*). *Commun. Behav. Biol.* 6:97–104.

Reese, T. S., and Brightman, M. W. 1970. Olfactory surface and central olfactory connexions in some vertebrates. *In* G. E. W. Wolstenholme and J. Knight (eds.). *Taste and Smell in Vertebrates.* J. and A. Churchill, London. Pp. 115–149.

Schaffer, J. 1940. *Die Hautdrüsenorgane des Säugertiere.* Urban and Schwarzenberg, Berlin.

Schilling, A. 1970. L'organe de Jacobson due lémurien malgache *Microcebus murinus* (Miller, 1777). *Mem. Mus. Nat. Hist. Nat. Ser. A Zool.* 61:203–280.

Schuckman, H., Kling, A., and Orbach, J. 1969. Olfactory discrimination in monkeys with lesions in the amygdala. *J. Comp. Physiol. Psychol. 67:*212–215.

Schultz, E. W. 1960. Repair of the olfactory mucosa. *Am. J. Pathol. 37:*1–19.

Seitz, E. 1969. Die Bedeutung geruchlicher Orientierung beim Plumplori, *Nycticebus coucang* Boddaert 1785 (*Prosimmii, Lorisidae*). *Z. Tierpsychol. 26:*73–103.

Shantha, T. R., and Nakajima, Y. 1970. Histological and histochemical studies on the rhesus monkey (*Macaca mulatta*). *Z. Zellforsch. Mikrosk. Anat. 103:*291–319.

Shantha Veerappa, T., and Bourne, G. 1965. Histochemical studies on the distribution of dephosphorylating and oxidative enzymes and esterases in the olfactory bulb of squirrel monkeys. *J. Nat. Cancer Inst. 35:*153–165.

Shantha Veerappa T., and Bourne G. H. 1966. Pacinian corpuscle on the olfactory bulb of the squirrel monkey. *Nature (London) 209:*1260.

Shepherd, G. M. 1972. Synaptic organization of the mammalian olfactory bulb. *Physiol. Rev. 52:*864–917.

Stephan, H. 1965. Der Bulbus olfactorius accessorius bei Insektivoren und Primaten. *Acta Anat. 62:*215–253.

Stephan, H., and Andy, O. J. 1969. Quantitive comparative neuroanatomy of primates: An attempt at a phytogenetic interpretation, *Ann. N.Y. Acad. Sci. 167:*370–387.

Tanabe, T., Iino, M., and Takagi, S. F. 1975a. Discrimination of odors in olfactory bulb, pyriform-amygdaloid areas, and orbitofrontal cortex of the monkey. *J. Neurophysiol. 38:*1248–1296.

Tanabe, T., Yarita, H., Iino, M., Ooshima, Y., and Takagi, S. F. 1975b. An olfactory projection area in orbitofrontal cortex of monkey. *J. Neurophysiol. 38:*1269–1283.

Vaccarezza, O. L., and Saavedra, J. P. 1968. Granulated vesicles in mitral cells and synaptic terminals of the monkey olfactory bulb. *Z. Zellforsch. Mikrosk. Anat. 87:*118–129.

Vinnikov, Y. A. 1956. Structure of the organ of smell. *Arkh. Anat. Gistol. Embriol. 33:*49–54.

von Holst, D. 1974. Social stress in the tree shrew: Its causes and physiological and ethological consequences. *In* R. D. Martin, G. A. Doyle, and A. C. Walker (eds.). *Prosimian Biology.* Gloucester Crescent, Duckworth. Pp. 389–411.

2

Physical and Physiological Principles Controlling Auditory Sensitivity in Primates

Shyam M. Khanna
and Juergen Tonndorf

I. Introduction

By way of introduction, we will give a brief description of the ear and the auditory nervous system. We will then discuss the role of the ear as an *early warning device*. The ear appears to be uniquely equipped for this role.

Traditionally, the mammalian ear is divided into three sections: the external, middle, and inner ears (Fig. 1). From the acoustical standpoint, the external and middle ears serve to protect the inner ear

SHYAM M. KHANNA AND JUERGEN TONNDORF • Department of Otolaryngology, College of Physicians and Surgeons, Columbia University, New York, New York 10027.

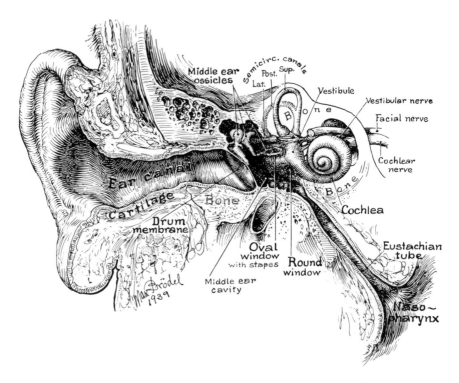

Fig. 1. Coronal cross section of a human ear on the right side. The section goes lengthwise through the external ear canal and through the middle ear. The inner ear, including the cochlea, is shown as if it were shelled out of the petrous bone; but it is presented in its correct anatomical position. The cochlear nerve is seen to enter the cochlea from the rear via the internal auditory canal. It is accompanied by the facial nerve and the vestibular nerve. (From Brödel, 1946.)

and to deliver to it a maximum of the incident acoustic energy. (This part of their function will be discussed in more detail later on.)

Acoustic energy entering the cochlear portion of the inner ear stimulates the specific sensory receptor cells, the hair cells of the organ of Corti. The acoustic (external) energy travels only up to this point. All responses elicited beyond it are manifestations of inherent biological forms of energy. Typical synapses are found between the hair cells and supplying sensory nerve fibers (Smith and Sjöstrand, 1961). Therefore, these fibers are most likely excited by the action of a chemical transmitter substance, although its exact nature is not yet known (Tonndorf, 1975). In the fibers of the cochlear nerve, the signal is transmitted in the form typical of all nerve fibers, that is, in the form of action potentials. These signals are transmitted along the neural pathways to reach eventually the auditory cortex (Fig. 2). They are processed at every one of the intermediate stations shown. This *afferent* (sensory) system is closely paralleled by an *efferent* system which acts as a feedback control on the auditory periphery (Rasmussen, 1946).

In man, the organ of Corti contains approximately 16,000 hair cells, about 3500 inner ones and 12,000 outer ones (Retzius, 1884). Structurally, the two types of hair cells differ slightly from each other

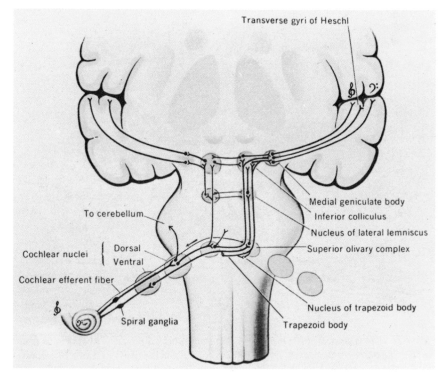

Fig. 2. The auditory pathways in man, schematically projected onto an outline of the brain and brainstem. Auditory nuclei begin in the spiral ganglion inside the modiolus and end at the auditory cortex, as shown. At every level, a tonotopic relationship exists, the basis of which is originally established by mechanical cochlear action. Note that the fibers from the two cochlear nuclei go to the nuclei of the superior olivary complex (specifically the accessory and the S-shaped nucleus) on *both* sides, indicating that these olivary nuclei receive ipsilateral as well as contralateral innervation. This is the first level of bilateral convergence, important for the analysis of binaurally received signals. (From Noback, 1967.)

(Fig. 3). They are distributed over the entire length of the cochlea in four parallel rows, one inner and three outer ones.

The afferent (sensory) innervation of the inner hair cells is strikingly different from that of the outer ones (Spoendlin, 1972). There are some 30,000 nerve fibers in man. About 90–95% of them supply the inner hair cells and the remaining 5–10% the outer ones. As shown in Fig. 4, each inner-hair-cell fiber runs out straight, i.e., "radially," from the modiolus and supplies only one cell; but each cell receives up to 20 such fibers. In contrast, the outer-hair-cell fibers run "longitudinally" for distances of approximately ½ mm in the direction of the cochlear

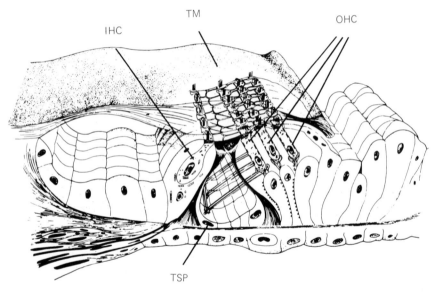

Figure 3.   Cross section of the organ of Corti, somewhat schematic. The modiolus is on the left, the outer cochlear wall on the right (both outside the picture frame). Shown are the single row of inner hair cells (IHC), the three rows of outer hair cells (OHC), and the tectorial membrane (TM), which hugs the organ rather tightly. The tips of the sensory cilia of each hair cell are embedded in this membrane. The afferent (radial) fibers supplying the inner hair cells are seen emerging from the habenula. The fibers supplying the outer hair cells actually have a more elaborate course than is shown here: (1) they are extremely fine fibers and run along the bottom of the tunnel space among the pillar-cell bodies, and are therefore hard to recognize; (2) they then course longitudinally for some distance before making connections to hair cells (for details of the innervation pattern, cf. Fig. 4). The fibers usually seen crossing through the middle of the tunnel, as in this figure, belong to the *efferent* system, as does the bundle of spiral tunnel fibers (TSP). (From Wersäll *et al.*, 1965.)

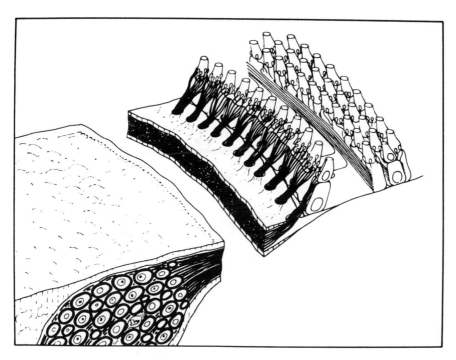

Fig. 4. Innervation pattern of cochlear hair cells (cat). Between 90 and 95% of all fibers run straight, i.e., "radially" to the inner hair cells (cf. Fig. 3), each fiber supplying only one cell, but each cell receiving up to 20 fibers. The fine-diameter fibers supplying the outer hair cells (5–10% of the total) originate from ganglion cells with lobulated nuclei (one of them is shown in the middle of the ganglion). After emerging from the habenula and crossing over the tunnel in the manner described in the legend to Fig. 3, these fibers run longitudinally toward the cochlear base for distances of approximately ½ mm and then supply 8–10 outer hair cells in a random fashion. (From Spoendlin, 1972.)

base before supplying about 10 outer hair cells in a completely random fashion. Hence, the patterns of supply of the two types of cells represent separately the principle of *divergence* (inner hair cells) and that of *convergence* (outer hair cells) of Sherrington.

Acoustic energy on reaching the cochlea rarely, if ever, stimulates all hair cells. There is a differentiation of frequency with place. High-frequency signals confine their stimulation to hair cells in the basal portion. As frequency is lowered, the place of stimulation moves gradually, and systematically, toward the cochlear apex (place principle of Helmholtz).

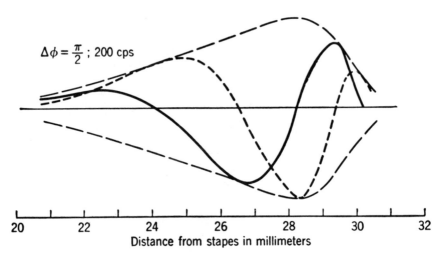

Fig. 5. Traveling-wave pattern for a frequency of 200 Hz in a human cadaver. Shown are two instances (the solid and the dashed waves) that are 90° apart in phase. Wave travel is from left to right; thus the solid wave represents the earlier instance of the two. Also given is the envelope (long dashed lines) delineating the long-term average of peak displacements. Note the gradual buildup toward a point of maximal displacement, the place of which is frequency-specific (at 28.3 mm for the present frequency), and the sharp decline of displacement amplitude beyond this point. (From Békésy, 1960.)

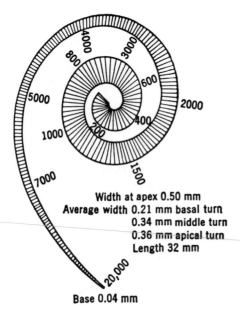

Width at apex 0.50 mm
Average width 0.21 mm basal turn
0.34 mm middle turn
0.36 mm apical turn
Length 32 mm

Base 0.04 mm

Fig. 6. Places of maximal displacement along the human basilar membrane for various frequencies as indicated. (Schematic from Stuhlmann, 1943.)

Fig. 7. Schematic presentation of one inner and three outer hair cells of the same cross-sectional plane viewed from the top. For further orientation, refer to Fig. 3. Note the typical W- or U-shaped patterns of stereocilia on the outer hair cells and the almost parallel pattern on the inner hair cell. It is only the tallest hairs in the outermost row on each cell that make contact with the tectorial membrane. The hairs decline in size with row number. Situated lateral to the stereocilia on each cell is the so-called basal body, the remnant of a tall thick hair that on cochlear hair cells is present only during embryological life. (It is a permanent feature of vestibular and lateral-line hair cells.) The fact that Held's drawing shows a small kinocilium on each cell instead of the basal body is an indication that he used embryological material. He may have done this because of the greater ease of preparation of the soft embryological bone that minimizes artifacts in unfixed material. Note that these details were observed by Held more than thirty years before the introduction of phase microscopy and forty years before the advent of scanning electron microscopy; both of these recent techniques confirmed his earlier findings in all details. (Adapted from Held, 1926.)

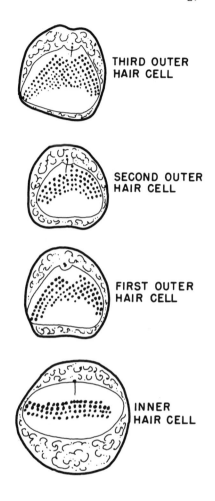

THIRD OUTER HAIR CELL

SECOND OUTER HAIR CELL

FIRST OUTER HAIR CELL

INNER HAIR CELL

This distribution of frequency along the cochlea is achieved mechanically by means of the *traveling-wave* phenomenon, first described by Békésy in 1928. That is to say, on stimulation of the cochlea a pattern of wavelike displacements moves along the cochlear duct from base to apex, forming frequency-dependent maxima in the manner just indicated (Fig. 5). Figure 6 shows in a somewhat schematic manner a frequency map of the human cochlea.

The displacements of the cochlear duct do not directly lead to a stimulation of hair cells. When the cochlear duct is displaced, a *shearing displacement* takes place between the organ of Corti and the tectorial membrane, and this in turn deflects the sensory cilia on top of the hair cells. It is this deflection that represents the ultimate mechanical input to the sensory cells. There are about 80–100 such cilia on each cell, arranged in characteristic patterns (Fig. 7).

The frequency-dependent distribution of the displacement maxima along the cochlear duct is the result of a mechanical *filtering* process; its cause is the traveling-wave mechanism. This becomes clear when one looks at the mechanical *tuning curve* of a given place along the cochlear duct. Figure 8 gives such a tuning curve obtained in squirrel monkey for a place near the basal end of the cochlea (Rhode, 1971). The frequency for which the response was maximal, the *best frequency*, was 8 kHz.

Tuning curves can also be obtained for single fibers of the cochlear nerve. Figure 9 gives a set of tuning curves in cat (Kiang *et al.*, 1965). The best frequencies of these tuning curves appear to be determined by the places along the cochlea at which the fibers connect with their hair cell(s).

A comparison of Figs. 8 and 9 indicates that the neural tuning curves are considerably sharper, by many orders of magnitude, than the mechanical ones. On the basis of a systematic comparison of this kind, Evans and Wilson (1973) proposed that the primary (mechanical) cochlear filter ought to be followed by a *second filter*.

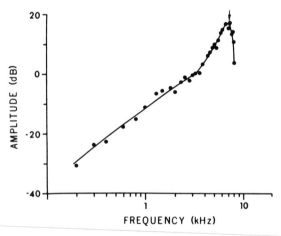

Fig. 8.   The mechanical tuning curve at a place close to the basal end of the basilar membrane of a squirrel monkey. Data were obtained with the aid of the Mössbauer technique. The frequency of maximal sensitivity, the "best frequency," of the place where the measurements were taken is 8 kHz. (From Rhode, 1971.)

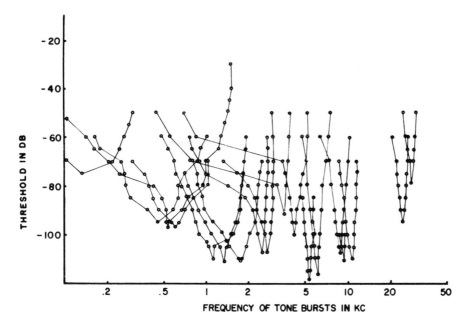

Fig. 9. A set of tuning curves of cochlear nerve fibers (cat) with different best frequencies. The points of maximal sensitivity at each best frequency follow approximately the cat's threshold curve. Compare the extreme sharpness of these neural tuning curves with that of the mechanical tuning curve of Fig. 8. (From Kiang *et al.*, 1965.)

This has been a rather condensed description, limited largely to points that will be of importance in the second part of the present chapter. More extensive descriptions of auditory function may be found in Békésy (1960), Dallos (1973), Green (1976), Tonndorf and Khanna (1976), and others.

II. The Ear as an Early Warning Device

The ear is a distance receptor, a distinction it shares with the eye and the sense of smell. Sound has a velocity that, although much slower than that of light, is still much faster than the speed of animal locomotion. The velocity of propagation of sound in air is 344 m/s and that in water 1500 m/s. The speed of even the fastest animal on land, in air, or in water is of the order of 20 m/s. The difference is such that the reception of acoustic signals, originating at some distance, occurs so early as to give the animal some time to react. Furthermore, sound transmission does not require a direct pathway between source and receiver.

By contrast, the sense of smell has to rely on the diffusion of molecules through the air or water, and that, compared to the speed of sound, is a rather slow process. The speed with which a light stimulus reaches the eye is faster by many orders of magnitude than that of a sound signal reaching the ear. This advantage is offset by several disadvantages: The passage of light requires a clear and direct pathway between the object and the eye, and vision depends on an adequate degree of illumination.

The advantages of sound just outlined indicate only the potential of an acoustic detector as an early warning device. How well such a detector can actually be adapted to this role depends on a number of features we must look at in more detail.

1. High Sensitivity of Detection. With increased distance, sound signals become greatly attenuated. Specifically, in a free field, i.e., in a space not bounded by large reflecting surfaces, sound intensity decreases with the square of the distance. This means that doubling the range of detection requires an increase in sensitivity by a factor of four. Clearly, there is a need for high sensitivity of detection, and the ear, as we shall presently see, is indeed a very sensitive detector.

2. Omnidirectional Reception. Variations of sensitivity with direction should be relatively minor. In particular, there should not be any dead zones which, for example, would allow a predator to close in on an animal from certain directions without the latter receiving a warning in time.

3. Localization of Sound Sources. When a sound is being received, it becomes important for the animal to assess the direction of its source of origin.

4. Detection of Sound in the Presence of Noise. In a real-life situation, the detection of acoustic signals invariably requires their differentiation against a background of noise.

In general, noises are sounds that have little, if any, useful information content. Thus, there is a need of noise reduction in order to assure optimal sensitivity.

5. Identification of the Sound Source. Once a sound is detected and its direction assessed, it becomes important to identify its source as quickly as possible from an analysis of its acoustic properties. It is only after this has been accomplished that the animal will be able to determine whether or not the sound is of any interest, i.e., whether it is a "signal" or may be disregarded. This is an important decision to make in view of the large number and variety of sensory inputs that, at any given time, impinge not only onto the auditory sense, but onto the other senses as well. Without such a sorting-out process, the central sensory receptors would be "jammed" most of the time. If the sound is of interest, the animal can decide on a deliberate course of action—closer inspection or escape, whichever might be indicated.

III. Sensitivity of Detection

As has already been mentioned, the usefulness of *any* detector depends on its sensitivity to the specific mode of energy to which it is responsive. Sensitivity may be maximized in two basic ways: (1) optimizing the delivery of energy to the detector either (i) by minimizing losses incurred on transmission to the detector, or (ii) by increasing the amount of energy collected from the environment; and (2) improving the detector's own performance.

A. Minimization of Transmission Losses

When an alternating (AC) signal such as sound impinges on a receiver, not all of the energy is necessarily admitted. The difficulty arises because the acoustic properties of the medium in which the energy travels and those of the receiver are not identical. Qualitatively, as well as quantitatively, the difference is best expressed in terms of *impedance*. Impedance may be defined in nonmathematical terms as the opposition of a medium to the flow of AC energy. The "characteristic" impedance of air to sound is low, i.e., 42 $dyn \cdot s \cdot cm^{-3}$; the "acoustic impedance of the fluid-filled inner ear is quite high, of the order of 10^6 $dyn \cdot s \cdot cm^{-5}$ (Khanna and Tonndorf, 1971; Lynch *et al.*, 1976).

Whenever such a *mismatch of impedance* exists, a large portion of the incoming energy is not transmitted to the receiver, but is reflected. Admission can be improved by *impedance matching*; this is accomplished by the interposition of a *transformer*. Under ideal circumstances, virtually 100% energy transmission can be achieved. A thorough discussion of impedance matching and of transformer action is beyond the scope of the present chapter. Their principles were first worked out in a formal manner in consideration of electrical networks. Reference must therefore be made to appropriate textbooks such as Pederson *et al.* (1966).

In the ears of mammals that receive acoustic energy from the surrounding air, the required impedance matching is achieved by a set of *mechanical* transformers consisting of the external and middle ears. In consequence of this transformer action, the sound pressure acting on the inner ear is increased relative to that existing in the surrounding air. The efficiency of the ear in this regard is quite high. (For details, see Békésy, 1960; Zwislocki, 1962, 1963; Tonndorf and Khanna, 1976.)

B. Increase in Energy Collection

Delivery of energy may also be improved, as has already been stated, by increasing the amount of energy collected by the receiver. This can be accomplished by enlarging its collecting surface, but this method is not without limitations.

To realize an increase in gain, the signal must arrive at an angle perpendicular to the plane of the receiving surface, so-called *normal incidence.* When the incidence is not normal, the amount of energy collected increases with the surface area up to a maximum, and beyond that it decreases again. This upper limit is given by the ratio of signal wavelength to the linear dimensions of the surface; it is reached when these dimensions approach ¼ wavelength. Since wavelength varies with frequency, the limit is frequency-dependent.

For an explanation, consider the spacing between subsequent fronts of condensation and rarefaction in a progressive acoustic wave (Fig. 10A); by definition, they are ½ wavelength apart. When the dimension of a surface exceeds ¼ wavelength, and when the wave front does not have normal incidence, condensations and rarefactions will act simultaneously on the receiving surface (Fig. 10B). They will thus partially, or even totally, cancel each other. As a result, the reception of energy becomes highly directional, the more so the larger the ratio between the dimension of the surface and ¼ wavelength.

Figure 11 shows a series of typical receiving patterns of this kind. Sensitivity is always maximal for normal incidence but decreases sharply as the angle of incidence is made larger. As is seen in Fig. 11, sharply defined minima may alternate with additional maxima,

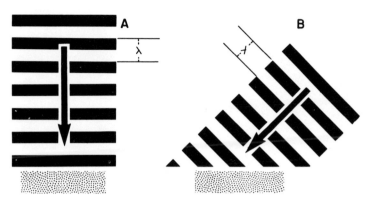

Fig. 10. A plane wave incident (A) normal to a vibrating surface, and (B) obliquely to the same surface. The wave consists of alternating compressions and rarefactions indicated by dark and light bands in the graphs. The spatial distance between any two consecutive full cycles is one wavelength (λ). (A) On normal incidence compressions or rarefactions act alternatingly on the surface. In this case, the force acting on the surface is directly proportional to the surface area. (B) On oblique incidence several compressions and rarefactions act simultaneously on the surface, as shown, thereby canceling each other's effects. The number of cycles of the wave that act on the surface simultaneously depends on the surface dimensions in terms of wavelength and on the angle of incidence. It is clear that perpendicular incidence will produce much larger vibration amplitudes than oblique incidence.

although the latter are always smaller in magnitude than the central maximum. The shorter the wavelength in relation to the dimensions of a given surface, the more complex the resulting pattern will be. Zones of good reception (maxima) alternate with virtual dead zones (minima). Therefore, an increase in the size of the receiving area will benefit only the reception of low frequencies.

In mammalian ears, reception of acoustic energy depends on its collection by the funnel composed of pinna and ear canal and on the size of the tympanic membrane. Figure 12 shows the relation between the area of the tympanic membrane in several classes of animals and the sensitivity of their ears at their most sensitive frequencies. The correlation could most likely be improved by also taking the effect of the pinna opening into account. Small animals tend to have relatively large pinnae.

It might also be of interest in this regard to learn how the size of the tympanic membrane varies with the body size of different animal species. Figure 13 shows that the area of the tympanic membrane changes with the cube root of the animal's body weight. In other words, the size of the tympanic membrane changes little as the body size varies over a large range.

C. Sensitivity of Biological Mechanodetectors

The sensitivity of biological mechanodetectors is far from uniform. It might be instructive to learn why some of them are more sensitive than others.

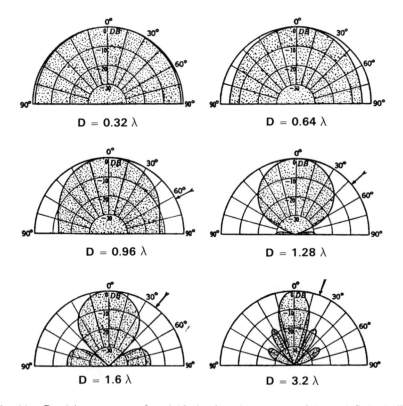

Fig. 11. Receiving patterns of a rigid circular piston mounted in an infinite baffle. When the dimensions of the receiving surface are small compared to the wavelength, the sound is received equally well from all frontal directions ($D = 0.32\ \lambda$). As dimensions are made larger in relation to the wavelength ($D = 0.64\ \lambda$ to $D = 3.2\ \lambda$), the receiving patterns become gradually directional. In these cases the sensitivity is highest for perpendicular incidence; it falls off sharply as the angle of incidence becomes smaller than 90°. See the legend of Fig. 10 for the cause of this directivity. (After Beranek, 1954.)

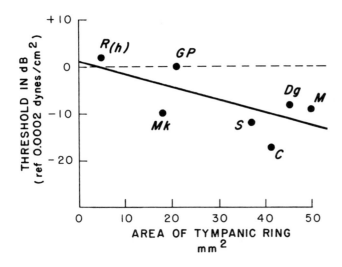

Fig. 12.   Auditory sensitivity at the best frequency as a function of area of the tympanic ring in a number of different animals ($R_{(h)}$, hooded rat; Mk, rhesus monkey; Gp, guinea pig; S, sheep; C, cat; Dg, dog; M, man). To a first approximation, the larger the receiving area, the higher will be the auditory sensitivity. A large number of additional factors influence sensitivity; they are discussed in the text.

Mechanoreceptors of the hair-cell type are found not only in the auditory organ, but also in two other phylogenetically related organs, the vestibular organs and the lateral-line organs of fishes and certain amphibia. In all of these organs the hair cells are connected to the sensory nerve endings by genuine synapses in the manner already described.

There is another class of mechanoreceptors. They consist simply of specialized receptor membranes on nerve endings upon which mechanical stimuli act directly. Such receptors then are *contact sensors*. Nerve spikes are generated when the mechanical deformation of the receptor membrane exceeds some threshold value. An example of such a receptor is the Pacinian corpuscle (Loewenstein, 1965).

These two types of mechanoreceptors differ vastly in sensitivity. The hair cells of vestibular and cochlear organs, for which reliable data are available (e.g., Oman and Young, 1972; Békésy, 1960), have sensitivities that are higher by very large factors, as much as 10^5, than those of receptors without hair cells. It has therefore been suggested that hair cells, in addition to their transducer task, act as *biological*

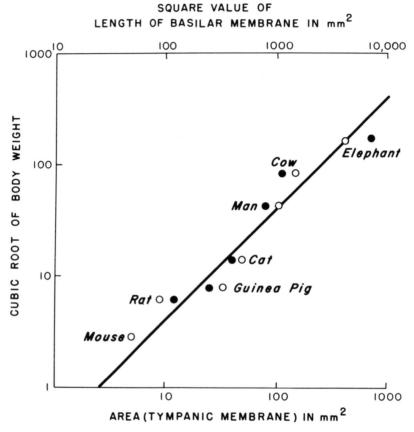

Fig. 13.   Area of the tympanic membrane (●) and the squared value of the length of the basilar membrane (O) vs. the cube root of body weight for several species. The area of the tympanic membrane varies roughly by a factor of 40 to 1 from the mouse to the elephant. (From Khanna and Tonndorf, 1968.)

amplifiers, a role for which they have apparently been specifically developed in order to improve sensitivity for the remote sensing of vibrations (Khanna, 1977).

IV. Directional Reception of Sound

Directional reception of sound, *auditory localization*, can be achieved to some degree by a single ear. However, it is mainly, and more accurately, accomplished by a central assessment of differences in the reception of the same sound by the two ears, i.e., by *binaural interaction*. Differences may be either in the sound pressure of the signal or in its time of arrival at the two ears; both of these vary systematically with the direction of the sound source in relation to the position of the animal's ears. *Interaural sound pressure differences* are important mainly for the localization of *high* frequencies and *interaural time differences* for that of *low* frequencies. Both of them result from purely acoustic causes.

A. Causes of Interaural Intensity Differences

The entire head casts an *acoustic shadow* that is sharper at higher frequencies since the effect is once more determined by the relation of head size to wavelength. Therefore, the ear on the side away from the sound source receives an attenuated signal.

The pinna is a directional receiver. However, on account of its highly asymmetrical shape, its receiving pattern is not as symmetrical as those shown in Fig. 11. Moreover, the characteristic folds and crevices of the pinna control the pattern with frequency in a highly predictable manner (Shaw, 1974). Figure 14 gives a polar diagram demonstrating, for a number of different frequencies, the directionality of a human ear in the horizontal plane, the combined result of head shadow and pinna effect. The higher the frequency the more pronounced is the directionality. Note that the reception of high frequencies is better from the front that from the rear on account of the shape of the pinna. Although not shown in Fig. 14, there are also variations of the receiving pattern with frequency in any other plane that can be laid through the axis of the ear canal, including the vertical (coronal) one.

The receiving patterns of the two ears in any plane from the horizontal to the vertical are mirror images of each other. It is seen therefore that for high frequencies the interaural pressure difference varies systematically with the position of a given sound source about the head. For sources that lie in the straight extension of the vertical (sagittal) midline through the head, the difference is extremely small.

When the signal is complex, the variations in directionality with frequency (Fig. 14) introduce *spectral* differences between the two ears. Again, these spectral differences exist in any plane from the horizontal to the vertical but, on account of the pinna effect, do not become zero

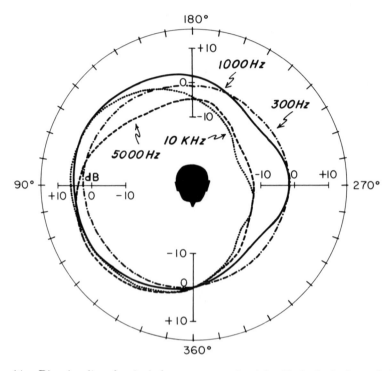

Fig. 14. Directionality of a single human ear on the right side in the horizontal plane at 300, 1000, 5000, and 10,000 Hz. The directionality is seen to increase at higher frequencies. (Based on data of Shaw, 1974.)

when the sound source lies in the extension of the vertical plane of the head. Spectral differences are of major importance for the localization of short-lasting ("transient") sounds with their *continuous*, wide-band, spectra. The briefer such transients, the farther their spectra extend into the high-frequency region.

B. Causes of Interaural Time Differences

Low frequencies with long wavelengths that exceed the dimensions of the head are diffused around it. Consequently, there is no head shadow, no pinna effect, and there are no appreciable interaural pressure differences either. However, when a low-frequency sound source is located on one side of the head, its distance from the two ears—and hence the travel time of the signal to them—is not the same, introducing an interaural time difference (Fig. 15). These time differences vary systematically with position in the horizontal plane, becoming once more very small when the source lies in the extension of the vertical midline plane through the head. For short-lasting clicks, the auditory system is able to detect extremely small interaural time differences of the order of 6 μs. For pure-tone signals, it is generally longer, more so for low frequencies than for high ones, e.g., 56 μs at 125 Hz and 11 μs at 1000 Hz.

Auditory localization, as was already mentioned, relies on interaural time differences for frequencies below approximately 1500 Hz in man and on interaural pressure differences for higher frequencies. The front-to-rear ambiguity in the horizontal plane (when both the time and intensity differences are zero) is resolved on the basis of spectral differences if the signal is a broad-band sound, as most naturally occurring signals are. Localization in the vertical plane relies mainly on spectral differences.

In small animals, the size of the head may be such that the interaural *time* differences are too brief for proper neurophysiological assessment. Consequently, this cue loses its value altogether. By the same token, the lowest frequency for which the head is able to cast an effective shadow must go up in value. Consequently, small animals appear to have a need for extended high-frequency hearing. Figure 16 gives the auditory high-frequency cutoff as a function of the maximal

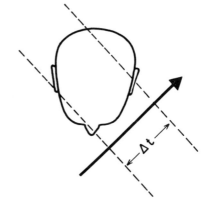

Fig. 15. When the sound source is located on one side of the head, the sound reaches the two ears at slightly different times. The magnitude of this interaural time difference is Δt. It varies with the position of the sound source around the head and the frequency.

interaural time difference for a number of animal species of various sizes. The interaural time difference is maximal for an angle of incidence of 90° (cf. Fig. 15). In man, its value is 630 μs. The smaller the head size, the smaller is the interaural time difference, and also the head shadow effect. Therefore, accuracy in localization can only be obtained at higher frequencies. Figure 18 shows that animals with small heads as a rule have extended high-frequency hearing.

Man achieves an accuracy in localizing a sound source in the horizontal plane of about ±1° around the sagittal midline of the head and of ±5° in the vertical plane. (Both values are again frequency dependent.) On any side of the midline, accuracy falls off rather sharply. This is the reason why animals, including man, on first receiving a sound turn their heads in the approximate direction of its source in an effort to improve accuracy if and when the sound is repeated. (For further details on directional hearing, see Green, 1976.)

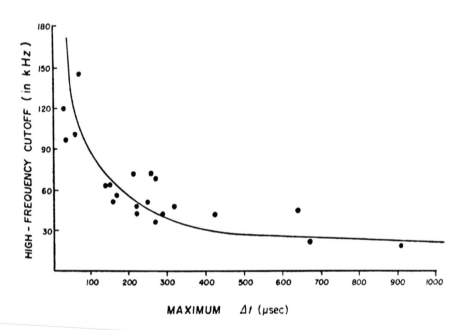

Fig. 16.   Auditory high-frequency cutoff as a function of maximal interaural time difference for a number of animal species of various sizes. Animals with smaller interaural time differences have extended auditory high-frequency ranges. (From Masterton and Diamond, 1973.)

Animals who are able to rotate their pinnae have an added advantage. Recall that for such a receiver, even a single one, intensity is maximal when the receiver is pointing directly toward the sound source (Fig. 11). Therefore, these animals rotate their pinnae in a scanning motion. Pointing the pinnae toward the source also aids in localization in the vertical plane. Dogs, for example, which are able to control the position of their pinnae, are much superior in this task compared to man, who is not able to do so.

C. Detection of Sound in the Presence of Noise

As was already stated, detectors as a rule must differentiate signals against a background of noise. Such noises may be of external or internal origin, and, as we shall see presently, they ultimately limit the sensitivity of the detector.

Pulsation of blood vessels, if present in the vicinity of cochlear hair cells, would, for example, stimulate these cells mechanically and thus limit their detection threshold. It is probably for that reason that no blood vessels run in close proximity to the cochlear hair cells (for details of cochlear blood supply, see Axelsson, 1968), and that their metabolic supply is by diffusion through the cochlear fluids (Vosteen, 1963).

V. Brownian Noise

Molecules of gases, fluids, and solids are constantly kept in motion by thermal agitation. This is known as Brownian motion, and its acoustic effect is *Brownian noise*. For example, the air molecules in front of the tympanic membrane randomly impinge on that membrane producing a, likewise random, stimulation of the ear. Harris (1968) calculated the noise level due to the Brownian noise of the air in front of the tympanic membrane. He found a level of 22 dB below the human auditory threshold. Recent calculations showed that, in the cat, the thermal noise level is at the threshold of hearing (Killion, personal communication), suggesting that the threshold value is determined mainly by noise.

VI. Improvement in Sensitivity of Detection by Reduction of Noise (Improvement of the Signal-to-Noise Ratio)

Although the noise level at the input to a given detector is not necessarily the only one affecting its threshold, we shall discuss this simple case first in order to make some general points.

If the bandwidth of the noise and that of the signal completely overlap, and if both of them are present at the same time, then the noise represents an irreducible limit below which detection of the signal is not possible. However, there are other situations in which the noise level may be reduced while the signal remains unaffected. If, for example, signal and noise are present simultaneously but occupy different frequency bands, the noise level can be reduced by means of *filters* with a resulting improvement in *signal-to-noise ratio*.

VII. The Effect of Narrow-Band Filters on Brownian Noise

Thermal (Brownian) noise is, by definition, uniformly distributed over all frequencies. The amount of noise energy that is being transmitted through a given filter depends entirely on the bandwidth of that filter. All frequencies outside the passband are rejected, and only those within it are transmitted. Therefore the total noise energy is attenuated in direct proportion to the reduced bandwidth.

Pure-tone signals represent a special case in this respect. The bandwidth of a pure tone is zero, if its frequency is held constant. Thus, narrowing the filter bandwidth will have no effect on signal transmission as long as the filter is centered around the signal frequency. In this case, narrow-band filtering can be employed to improve the signal-to-noise ratio to an almost unlimited extent.

In contrast, real-life signals such as speech do not have constant frequencies but vary continually and rather rapidly with time. (Nonvarying signals would not be able to carry any information.) Variations in frequency imply that the signal stays for only limited time intervals within the bandwidth of a given filter.

As the signal sweeps into the passband of the filter, the filter output does not instantly rise to its ultimate value. It builds up slowly with time. This *rise time* is inversely proportional to the filter bandwidth. For example, the rise time of a simple filter with a bandwidth of 100 Hz is approximately $k/100$ s; the constant k has a value of about 0.4 (Terman and Pettit, 1952). Therefore, the output of such a filter will never attain its full value if the signal stays within the filter bandwidth for less than $1/250$ s. In this case, a filter with a wider bandwidth would yield a higher output.

We may look at another aspect of this problem. If the ear were to employ filters of very narrow bandwidths and if the signal to be detected were barely above threshold, the prolonged rise time would in effect introduce a long time delay until the signal finally became audible. A long delay of this kind might prove fatal for the animal in question.

There is another factor, and that is also related to the bandwidth of the filters in the ear. It has to do with the information-carrying capacity of single auditory nerve fibers. Their maximal firing rate is of the order of 200 spikes/s. General sampling theory predicts that under such a condition the maximal signal frequency that may be transmitted is approximately 100 Hz. If, however, the bandwidths of the filters preceding the nerve fibers were narrower than this value, the information-carrying capacity of the fibers would not be fully utilized. These considerations indicate that the bandwidths of the filters employed by the ear may be narrowed only to a limit, but that further reduction beyond that limit would be disadvantageous for the overall function.

Table I has been prepared from the tuning curves of auditory nerve fibers as presented in Fig. 9. It shows the estimated average bandwidth of these fibers to be of the order of 100 Hz.

TABLE I.   Estimated 3 dB Bandwidths and Rise Times Derived from the Tuning Curves of the Primary Auditory Fibers[a]

Center frequency (Hz)	Estimated 3 dB bandwidth (Hz)	Approximate rise time (sec)
0.5	60	7×10^{-3}
2.0	134	3×10^{-3}
10.0	232	1.75×10^{-3}

[a] Based on data from Kiang *et al.* (1965).

VIII. Detection of Signals

After the signal-to-noise ratio has been improved by narrow-band filtering, a detector is required at the end of each filter to determine if a signal was in fact present at the filter input.

Optimal detection requires one detector for each filter. If the detector were connected to more than one filter, it would receive noise from each of them. This would lessen its sensitivity and defeat the whole purpose of the narrow-band filtering.

The simplest type of its kind is a *threshold detector*. Such a device produces an output pulse whenever a signal exceeds a given threshold value. If noise is present within the system, some of its peaks may occasionally exceed the threshold value, each producing an output pulse even though a signal was not actually present at the input. In the parlance of signal detection theory (Green and Swets, 1966), this is known as a "false alarm."

If the threshold of the detector were set so high as to avoid the occurrence of false alarms altogether, signals would have to be raised proportionally before they could be detected. This would render the detector rather insensitive. What is obviously needed in such a case is to find a compromise between sensitivity and the number of false alarms that can be tolerated.

One of the inherent properties of simple threshold detectors is their narrow dynamic range. That is to say, the firing rate reaches its maximal value as soon as the signal exceeds the threshold of the detector.

The method of detection actually employed by the auditory system appears to be much more complex than that of the simple threshold detector just described. Figure 17 gives the firing rates of auditory nerve fibers as a function of signal intensity. When the signal is below the threshold of detection (or when there is no signal present) there are spontaneous, random discharges. As the signal intensity exceeds the threshold value, the firing rate increases, to reach eventually a peak value; beyond that, it decreases again. In some fibers, the firing rate keeps increasing over a range as wide as 40 dB, and, after reaching its maximum, it keeps decreasing continuously for another 40 dB, making a total range of 80 dB, and sometimes an even wider one. Such a wide range of responses could be brought about either (a) by letting the threshold of the detector be dynamically altered ("adapted") by the level

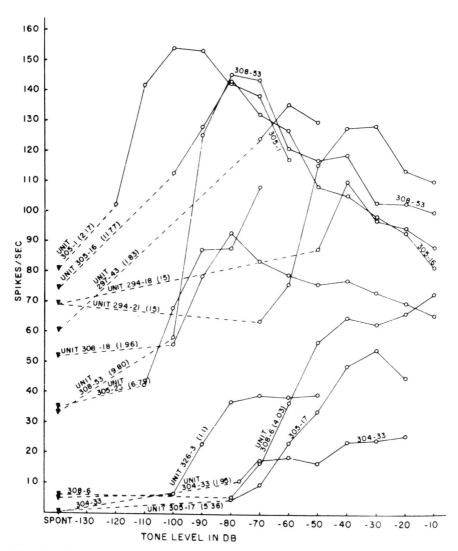

Fig. 17.   Rate of firing as a function of the level of the tone. For each curve, data were
obtained at the center frequency of the auditory nerve fiber (cat) in question. When no
sound is present, fibers fire at some spontaneous rates. As tone level is raised, the firing
rate increases and then reaches a peak. Further increases in level beyond that point let
the curve either level off or decrease again. (From Kiang *et al.*, 1965.)

of the signal, or (b) by letting the gain of the system preceding the detector be controlled by the input level.

If it is correct that the sensitivity of the detector in the auditory system is limited by the noise, a detector of high sensitivity ought to have a threshold close to the noise. It should therefore have a high rate of spontaneous activity. Recent measurements have indeed demonstrated a good correlation between the spontaneous discharge rate of cochlear nerve fibers and their sensitivity (Kiang *et al.*, 1976).

IX. Multiple Sources of Noise

As has already been stated, not all of the noise that may act upon a given detector system exists exclusively at the input. In that situation, it is relatively easy to predict the statistics of the noise as it appears at the output of the filter. (Random noises can only be defined in statistical terms.) A more complex situation arises (a) when there is more than one source of noise in the system, (b) when the noise statistics differ among the various sources, (c) when these noises are introduced at different levels of the system so that each of them is affected differently by the filtering process, and (d) when there is more than one filter connected in series, each of a different characteristic.

In addition to the Brownian noise source in front of the tympanic membrane that has already been mentioned, other sources of noise may exist (a) in the fluids of the inner ear, (b) in the mechanical structures of the organ, (c) in the amplification process in hair cells, and (d) in the events associated with synaptic transmission (Schroeder and Hall, 1974). The statistics of the two last-named noises are likely to differ from those of the others because their mechanisms of production are different.

If the Brownian noise at the tympanic membrane were the dominant source of noise in the auditory organ, the spontaneous activity of simple nerve fibers should reflect the response to such an input as seen through the appropriate cochlear filter. Therefore, the level of spontaneous activity should be higher for fibers with large bandwidths and vice versa. No such relationship has been demonstrated (Kiang *et al.*, 1965). This finding supports the general notion of multiple cochlear noise sources and, in particular, the assumption that some of them must be located beyond the cochlear filters, i.e., either in the hair cells or in the hair cell–nerve junction.

Each filter–detector channel of the peripheral auditory system has a rather narrow bandwidth (see Fig. 9); in the cat, according to Table I, it varies between 60 Hz and 250 Hz. A complete coverage of the total range of hearing requires a *parallel array* of a large number of such channels. The question is: how many channels in parallel are needed? If the total range to be covered is B, and if the average bandwidth of the individual filters is b (both given in hertz), then B/b is the required minimum. In other words, the narrower the bandwidth b or the wider the total frequency range B, the more individual filters are needed.

The mechanical tuning along the basilar membrane varies in a *continuous* manner. Thus, this system does not employ discrete filters. Discrete channels first come into being at the hair-cell level and continue to exist in the individual fibers of the cochlear nerve.

The total auditory range of cats is about 40,000 Hz. With an average bandwidth of about 100 Hz then, a minimum of 400 filter channels and detectors (hair cells) are needed. However, the combined output of these 400 channels would not be smooth. There would be drops in sensitivity of about 3 dB every 100 Hz. With about 800 channels there would be more overlap, and the overall response would be smooth within 1 dB. In cat, the total number of hair cells available is very much larger, 2600 inner hair cells and 9900 outer ones (Retzius, 1884) than the minimum needed for sensitive detection of signals. Why the number is that large is not understood at this time.

X. Concluding Remarks

The present chapter discussed a number of general principles involved in the reception of sound and its detection. The physical dimensions of the head and those of the ear were shown to be significant in determining the performance of the auditory system. Some of these dimensions must clearly be the result of a compromise between conflicting requirements: (a) to collect an optimal amount of acoustic energy over a wide range of frequencies; (b) to avoid the creation of dead zones in the directional pattern of hearing; (c) to facilitate auditory localization both in the horizontal plane and in the vertical one.

Sensitivity is close to its optimal value, i.e., it is essentially determined by the noise in the system itself. Figure 18 presents threshold sensitivity vs. frequency for a number of representative primates. It is seen that among these animals the sensitivity at the best fre-

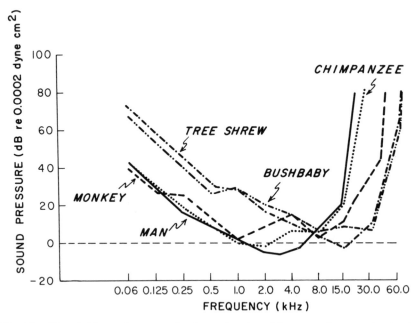

Fig. 18. Threshold sound pressure level as a function of frequency for several primates (man, monkey, chimpanzee, bushbaby, and tree shrew). Sensitivities at the best frequencies are within 10 dB of each other. (Adapted from Stebbins, 1971.)

quency varies by not more than 10 dB, i.e., by a relatively small amount, although the relationship originally presented in Fig. 12 can once more be recognized. The high-frequency cutoff varies inversely with the size of the head, supporting the conclusion expressed in connection with Fig. 16, i.e., that small animals need extended high-frequency hearing for the purpose of auditory localization. The low-frequency end shows an opposite trend. This is related to the fact, shown in Fig. 13, that the area of the tympanic membrane is a function of body size. However, as the tympanic membrane area is made larger and low-frequency reception is improved, reception of high frequencies must be reduced. This might explain why in Fig. 18 the width of the auditory range stays approximately constant when frequency is plotted logarithmically in the usual manner. That is to say, the ratio between the cutoff at high frequencies and that at low frequencies is about the same for all species.

The present discussion never goes beyond the confines of the ear. However, central auditory processing just *begins* there. It is continued on each subsequent level from the cochlear nuclei up to the cortex. For example, the signal-to-noise ratio is further enhanced, a task that is aided by the action of the efferent auditory system and, under some conditions, also by binaural interactions. The auditory cortex plays a decisive role in sound localization and in the recognition of the temporal patterns of sound (Neff *et al.*, 1975). These and other central auditory functions are beyond the scope of the present chapter.

XI. References

Axelsson, A. 1968. The vascular anatomy of the cochlea in the guinea pig and in man. *Acta Oto-Laryngol. Suppl.* 243.

Békésy, G. von, 1960. *Experiments in Hearing.* E. G. Wever (trans. and ed.). McGraw-Hill, New York.

Beranek, L. L. 1954. *Acoustics.* McGraw-Hill, New York.

Brödel, M. 1946. *Three Unpublished Drawings of the Anatomy of the Human Ear.* W. B. Saunders, Philadelphia.

Dallos, P., 1973, *The Auditory Periphery.* Academic Press, New York.

Evans, E. F., and Wilson, J. P. 1973. Frequency selectivity of the cochlea. *In* A. Møller (ed.). *Basic Mechanisms in Hearing.* Academic Press, New York. Pp. 519–551.

Green, D. M. 1976. *An Introduction to Hearing.* John Wiley, New York.

Green, D. M., and Swets, J. A. 1966. *Signal Detection Theory and Psychophysics.* John Wiley, New York.

Harris, G. G. 1968. Brownian motion in the cochlear partition. *J. Acoust. Soc. Am.* 44:176–186.

Held, H. 1926. Die Cochlea der Säuger und der Vögel, ihre Entwicklung und ihr Bau. *In* A. Bethe (ed.). *Handbuch der normalen und pathologischen Physiologie,* II, *Receptionsorgane* I. Springer, Berlin. Pp. 467–534.

Khanna, S. M. 1977. Unpublished data.

Khanna, S. M., and Tonndorf, J. 1968. Middle ear power transfer. *Arch. Klin. Exp. Ohren. Nasen. Kehlkopfheilk.* 193:78–88.

Khanna, S. M., and Tonndorf, J. 1971. The vibratory pattern of the round window in cats. *J. Acoust. Soc. Am.* 50:1475–1483

Kiang, N. Y. S., Watanabe, T., Thomas, E. C., and Clark, L. F. 1965. Discharge patterns of single fibers in the cat's auditory nerve. *MIT Research Monograph* No. 35. MIT Press, Cambridge, Mass.

Kiang, N. Y. S., Liberman, M. C., and Levine, R. A. 1976. Auditory nerve activity in cats exposed to ototoxic drugs and high intensity sounds. *Ann. Otol. Rhinol. Laryngol. 75:* 752–768.

Loewenstein, W. R. 1965. Facets of a transducer process. *In Cold Spring Harbor Symposia on Quantitive Biology,* Vol. XXX, *Sensory Receptors.* Cold Spring Harbor Laboratory of Quantitative Biology, Cold Spring Harbor, L.I., N.Y. Pp. 29–43.

Lynch, T. J., III, Nedzelnitsky, V., and Peake, W. T. 1976. Measurements of acoustic input impedance of the cochlea in cats (A). *J. Acoust. Soc. Am. 59,* Suppl. 30.

Masterton, B., and Diamond, I. T. 1973. Hearing: Central neural mechanisms. *In* (E. C. Carterette and M. P. Friedman, eds.). *Handbook of Perception*, Vol. III. Academic Press, New York.

Neff, W. D., Diamond, I. T., and Casseday, J. H. 1975. Behavioral studies of auditory discrimination. *In* W. D. Keidel and W. D. Neff (eds.). *Handbook of Sensory Physiology*, Vol. 2. *Auditory System*. Springer, New York. Pp. 307–400.

Noback, C. R., 1967. *The Human Nervous System*. McGraw-Hill, New York.

Oman, C. M., and Young, L. R. 1972. The physiological range of pressure difference and cupula deflections in the human semicircular canal. *Acta Oto-Laryngol.* 74;324–331.

Pederson, D. O., Studer, J. J., and Whinnery, J. 1966, *Introduction to Electronic Systems, Circuits and Devices*. McGraw-Hill, New York.

Rasmussen, G. L. 1964. The olivary peduncle and other fiber projections of the superior olivary complex. *J. Comp. Neurol.* 84:141–219.

Retzius, G. 1884. *Das Gehörorgan der Wirbeltiere*, Vol. II. *Das Gehörorgan der Reptilien, der Vögel, und der Säugetiere*. Samson and Wallin, Stockholm.

Rhode, W. S. 1971. Observations of the vibration of the basilar membrane in squirrel monkeys using the Mössbauer technique. *J. Acoust. Soc. Am.* 49:1218–1231.

Schroeder, M. R., and Hall, J. L. 1974. Model for mechanical to neural transduction in the auditory receptor, *J. Acoust. Soc. Am.* 55:1055–1060.

Shaw, E. A. G. 1974. The external ear. *In* W. D. Keidel and W. D. Neff (eds.). *Handbook of Sensory Physiology*, Vol. V/1. Springer, New York. Pp. 455–490.

Smith, C. A., and Sjöstrand, F. S. 1961. A synaptic structure in the hair cells of the guinea pig cochlea. *J. Ultrastruct. Res.* 5:184–192.

Spoendlin, H. 1972. Innervation densities of the cochlea. *Acta Oto-Laryngol.* 73:235–248.

Stebbins, W. C. 1971. Hearing. *In* A. M. Schrier and F. Stollnitz (eds.). *Behaviour of Non-Human Primates*, Vol. III. Academic Press, New York. Pp. 159–192.

Stuhlmann, O., Jr. 1943. *An Introduction to Biophysics*. John Wiley, New York.

Terman, F. E. and Pettit, J. M. 1952. *Electronic Measurements*. McGraw-Hill, New York.

Tonndorf, J. 1975. Davis—1961 Revisited. *Arch. Otolaryngol.* 101: 528–535.

Tonndorf, J., and Khanna, S. M. 1976. Mechanics of the auditory system. *In* R. Hinchcliffe and Harrison, D. (eds.). *Scientific Foundations of Otolaryngology*. William Heinemann, London. Pp. 237–252.

Vosteen, K. H. 1963. New aspects in the biology and pathology of the inner ear, *Transl. Beltone Inst. Hear. Res.* 16:1–30.

Wersäll, J., Flock, A., and Lundquist, P. G. 1965. Structural basis for directional sensitivity in cochlear and vestibular sensory receptors. *In Cold Spring Harbor Symposia on Quantitative Biology*, Vol. XXX, *Sensory Receptors*. Cold Spring Harbor Laboratory of Quantitative Biology, Cold Spring Harbor, L.I., N.Y. Pp. 115–132.

Zwislocki, J. 1962. Analysis of the middle ear function. Part I. Input impedance. *J. Acoust. Soc. Am.* 34:1514–1523.

Zwislocki, J. 1963. Analysis of the middle ear function. Part II. Guinea-pig ears. *J. Acoust. Soc. Am.* 35:1034–1040.

3

The Anatomical Organization of the Primate Auditory Pathways

Norman L. Strominger

I. Introduction

The mammalian auditory pathway consists of several nuclear complexes and interconnecting fiber tracts extending between the receptors located in the cochlea and the cerebral cortex. Bipolar perikarya of the primary neurons form the spiral ganglion and are part of the peripheral nervous system. Well-defined nuclei in the central nervous system include the cochlear nuclei, superior olivary complex, ventral nucleus of the lateral lemniscus, dorsal nucleus of the lateral lemniscus, inferior colliculus, medial geniculate body, and the auditory areas of the cerebral cortex.

Norman L. Strominger • Department of Anatomy, Albany Medical College of Union University, Albany, New York 12208. Supported in part by NIH Grants HS-06350 and NS-12208.

There are more nuclei in the auditory system and the pathway is more complicated than in other sensory systems. There also is an additional mandatory synapse in the auditory pathway of nonprimates and of primates at least through the phylogenetic level of *Macaca mulatta*; a minimum of four neurons, rather than three as in other sensory pathways, constitute the chain from the periphery to the cerebral cortex for most mammals. A common explanation for the unusual nature of the auditory pathway is based upon the late development of hearing in phylogenesis. Because of this, the auditory pathway presumably incorporated scattered structures which still were modifiable in what already had become a relatively stable nervous system. Another reason concerns the nature of audition itself. Hearing involves the analyses of such diverse functions as intensity, frequency, pattern, distance, direction, etc., and may perforce require a more complex pathway than other sensory systems.

Although a voluminous literature exists concerning the neuroanatomical substrate as well as the behavioral and physiological mechanisms of audition, most information about the anatomy of the auditory pathways has been derived from experiments with nonprimates. Understanding of the human auditory system is based largely upon extrapolations from these studies.

What follows is a description of the auditory pathways. Wherever possible this is based on studies done with primates, but because the exposition would be incomplete otherwise, and for historical perspective, numerous references are made to experiments done with other mammals, notably the cat.

II. Morphological Aspects of the Auditory Pathway

A. Cochlear Nuclei

1. Subdivisions. The cochlear complex consists of two main divisions referred to as the dorsal and ventral cochlear nuclei. The latter is subdivided into anteroventral and posteroventral cochlear nuclei. While it is possible on a cytoarchitectural basis to subdivide the complex further, the dorsal anteroventral and posteroventral cochlear nuclei appear to be functionally important major subdivisions. Rose *et al.* (1959, 1960), using the cat, demonstrated that each subdivision is tonotopically organized. There is an orderly progression of neurons within each subdivision in a dorsoventral sequence which are maximally sensitive to sound stimuli from high to low frequencies respectively. Thus, the auditory frequency spectrum is represented by neural units at three different loci at the level of the cochlear nuclei. A multiple representation of the cochlea is a characteristic feature of the auditory system.

2. Neuronal Population. Based on microscopic analyses of Nissl preparations, nine distinct perikaryal types have been enumerated in the cochlear complex of the cat (Osen, 1969), viz., small spherical cell, large spherical cell, globular cell, multipolar cell, small cell, octopus cell, pyramidal cell, giant cell, and granule cell. According to their distribution, the cochlear complex was divided into separate though partially overlapping cell areas. Brawer *et al.* (1974) prepared a cytoarchitectonic atlas of the cat cochlear complex and plotted on outline drawings the position of individual cells determined by observations of Golgi material. These investigators categorized twenty cell types using morphological properties of the perikarya together with the axons and dendrites. Some of the types thus described may represent variants of a single perikaryal category. The present scheme of organization of the primate cochlear complex is based on observations of Nissl-stained sections and undoubtedly will be elaborated upon when Golgi studies are completed.

Several cell types corresponding to most of those described by Osen (1969) can be distinguished in the rhesus monkey and the human. Granule cells may be absent from the human cochlear complex. Giant cells are rare in the rhesus monkey and inconstant in the human. According to Moscowitz (1969), they are not evident in the squirrel monkey or several other primates. Further, in the macaque and man, there is no dichotomy between small and large spherical cells (Strominger and Strominger, 1971; Bacsik and Strominger, 1973). Perikarya, with usually an ovoid contour corresponding in locations to the spherical types described by Osen, form a single population with respect to area, though there is a considerable range in size. Moreover, larger and smaller perikarya are spatially intermixed. Some of the cells intermixed with the ovoid perikarya are spherical in shape. It was assumed because of common cytoarchitectural features that this was a function of the plane of section and variation in contour. It deserves mention that large and small spherical cells have been differentiated in the squirrel monkey (Moscowitz and Liu, 1972); it may or may not be relevant that this species is a New World monkey.

While different parts of the cochlear complex may be characterized by the presence of a given cell type, no one area is the exclusive domain of a single perikaryal population. The borders between the chief cell types and subdivisions appear less sharp than described in the cat. Also, in Nissl preparations, a certain percentage of the cells cannot be classified reliably. Occasionally, a cell readily assigned to a category will be found far removed from others of this type. The following description of the subdivisions of the cochlear complex considers some of the main features and is not meant to include all the fine details of its organization.

   3. The Anteroventral Cochlear Nucleus.   The anteroventral cochlear nucleus (Av) forms the rostral part of the cochlear complex. Toward the oral pole, it is situated between the root of the vestibular nerve and the peduncle of the flocculus (Fig. 1). The cochlear root is present at caudal levels along the ventral and medial aspects of the nucleus.

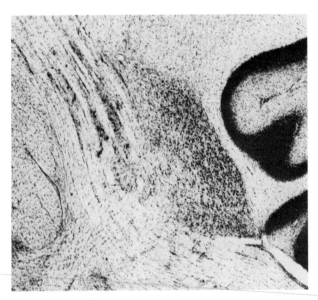

Fig. 1. Photomicrograph of transverse section near the oral end of the right anteroventral cochlear nucleus of the rhesus monkey. The vestibular root borders Av ventrally and medially at this level. Parts of the flocculus and spinal trigeminal tract appear at the right and left of the micrograph respectively. Cresyl violet, ×20.

Ovoid cells, perhaps a more appropriate designation in primates for the spherical type, occupy the bulk of the Av, extending caudally from its oral pole. They are densely packed orally and somewhat less compactly arranged at caudal levels due to the presence of a greater number of entering primary fibers which pass in a rostral direction. Small cells occasionally intermingle with the much more conspicuous oval neurons and are found throughout the cochlear complex. Some multipolar cells, embracing a variety of multangular forms and probably cell types, also may be present along the medial border at all but the oral pole of the Av; perikarya of this nature also have a widespread distribution. The ovoid cell type is absent toward the caudal end of the Av. Globular cells, the characteristic but not exclusive type here, extend into the region of entry of the cochlear root and immediately behind it. This represents a blurring of the boundary between the anteroventral and posteroventral cochlear nuclei. The globular perikarya typically have a plump oval contour with a markedly eccentric nucleus which frequently forms a bulge along one side of the cell. Ovoid cells also tend to have an eccentric nucleus, but the eccentricity is less marked and does not cause a bulge. The globular cells also have finer Nissl particles. The distinction between ovoid and globular cells is greater in the rhesus monkey than in the human.

4. The Posteroventral Cochlear Nucleus. The posteroventral cochlear nucleus (Pv) begins at the level of entrance of the cochlear root into the brain stem and continues to the caudal tip of the cochlear complex where it is capped posteriorly by the dorsal cochlear nucleus (Fig. 2).

Multipolar cells are concentrated in the rostral end of Pv. Toward the caudal end of this subdivision of the cochlear complex, octopus cells are characteristic though not present in large numbers. Octopus cells are more or less shield-shaped in full profile with processes emitted at the three apices. Most often the perikarya are somewhat rotated and present a crescentic appearance, which makes them more difficult to identify. It should be noted that all the cell types mentioned thus far are more readily identified in the rhesus monkey than in the human. In the latter, classification of a much greater number of individual neurons becomes uncertain with the Nissl stain. Poorer postmortem preservation of cells at least partially accounts for the problem.

5. The Dorsal Cochlear Nucleus. The dorsal cochlear nucleus (DCN), located at the junction between the medulla and pons, forms a

prominent tubercle at the posterolateral aspect of the brainstem between
the inferior cerebellar peduncle and the flocculus (Fig. 3). The dorsal
surface underlies part of the floor of the lateral recess of the fourth
ventricle. Caudally, the DCN presents free lateral and posterior surfaces
in the macaque; its posterior pole may be confused with the pontobulbar
nucleus which covers it in man. Orally, neurons of this nucleus
interdigitate with those of the Av. The DCN generally covers the
posteroventral subdivision along its dorsolateral aspect. The DCN was
described by Ramón y Cajal (1909) as being poorly developed in the
human and is considered relatively reduced in primates, including man
(Olszewski and Baxter, 1954; Stotler, 1957; Moscowitz, 1969).

One of the striking features of the dorsal cochlear nucleus is its distinct lamination in some species, of which the cat is a good example. In

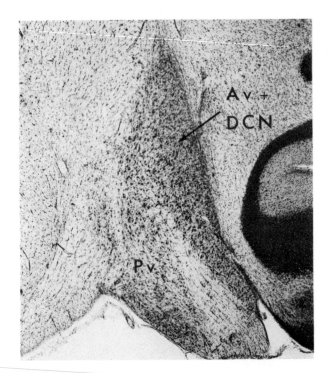

Fig. 2.   Photomicrograph of transverse section near the rostral end of the right
posteroventral cochlear nucleus of the rhesus monkey. At this level, the cochlear root
partially separates the posteroventral nucleus (Pv) from a transitional region containing
perikarya characteristic of both the anteroventral (Av) and dorsal (DCN) cochlear
nuclei. Cresyl violet, ×20.

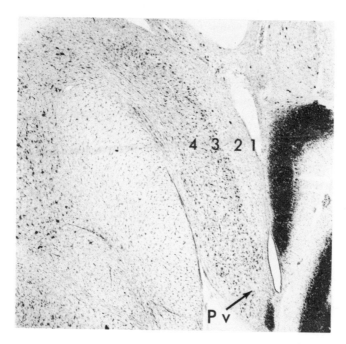

Fig. 3. Photomicrograph of a transverse section near the caudal end of the right dorsal cochlear nucleus of the rhesus monkey showing its lamination into: (1) epithelial, (2) molecular, (3) pyramidal, and (4) polymorphic layers. The posteroventral cochlear nucleus (Pv) is at the bottom of the photomicrograph. The flocculus is to the right and the inferior cerebellar peduncle to the left of the cochlear nuclei. Cresyl violet, ×20.

addition to a surface epithelium, molecular (outer plexiform), pyramidal (granular), and polymorphic (inner plexiform) layers are recognized. The distinctness of this laminar organization is variable within the primate order. It is quite clear in the rhesus monkey, and somewhat obscure in the human DCN. In the former, scattered granule cells characterize the molecular layer. These small neurons with scant cytoplasm impart a lightly staining appearance to the layer in Nissl-stained sections. Somewhat larger neurons are occasional constituents. The pyramidal cells, for which the next layer is named, are fusiform elements oriented perpendicular or obliquely to the surface of the complex. This layer of conspicuous cells gives the DCN its characteristic appearance in species where the DCN is distinctly laminated. While their orientation remains the same in the rhesus monkey, the perikarya no longer are aligned so neatly in a level array. Instead, pyramidal cells extend into the polymorphic layer, and these two laminae are not so sharply delimited. There is some variability in this regard in different animals and at different levels.

The presence of granule cells is questionable in the human, yet some degree of lamination is evident. The pyramidal cells now are oriented with their long axes parallel to the surface as noted by Olszewski and Baxter (1954) (Fig. 4).

The polymorphic layer, or central part of the DCN, contains a diverse population of cells, including small cells, pyramidal cells, and multipolar cells. Giant-type perikarya are rare but constant constituents in the rhesus monkey and chimpanzee. Two or three neurons of this

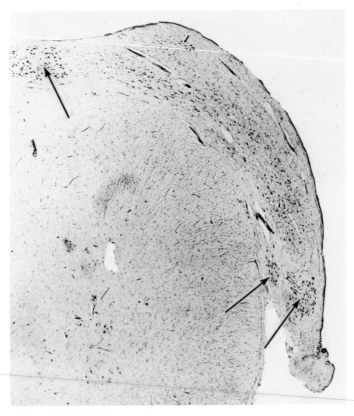

Fig. 4.   Photomicrograph of transverse section of the human dorsal cochlear nucleus on the right side. Some degree of lamination is evident. Arrows point to perikarya of the pontobulbar nucleus. Cresyl violet, ×20.

type have been seen in some but not all human brainstems. Considering that every section through the DCN is not stained, it is estimated that there are 0–15 giant cells. The reasons for the changes in anatomical organization of the dorsal cochlear nucleus have not be elucidated.

B. Superior Olivary Complex

The superior olivary comlex is the most caudal level of the auditory pathway at which ascending fiber systems issuing from the two sides converge. Binaural interaction in the superior olivary complex is important to the mechanisms of sound localization and other phenomena. The complex, located in the ventral part of the caudal pontine tegmentum of primates, is comprised of several subnuclei. These are designated the lateral superior olivary nucleus (SOL), medial superior olivary nucleus (SOM), nucleus of the trapezoid body, lateral preolivary nucleus, medial preolivary nucleus, and the periolivary cell groups.

1. Lateral Superior Olivary Nucleus. The name superior olive is derived from the lateral segment which in carnivores has an S-shaped configuration and is the most conspicuous component. For this reason it sometimes is referred to as the principal or main nucleus or simply the superior olive proper. However, this terminology cannot be applied to primates where the SOL is said to regress.

The lateral superior olive of the rhesus monkey is essentially oval in shape with slight dorsal and ventral indentations (Fig. 5). The outline of the segment is variable in different primates as illustrated by Moscowitz (1969) and Moore and Moore (1971). Although some investigators have considered the SOL to be rudimentary in the human (Papez, 1930; Stotler, 1953; Olszewski and Baxter, 1954), studies by Moore and Moore (1971) and recently in my laboratory (Strominger and Hurwitz, 1976) have demonstrated that it contains a substantial neuronal population (see Fig. 6). Our data indicate that there is an average of roughly 3900 perikarya in the human SOL. The segment is inconspicuous because it is composed of as many as five separate clusters of cells rather than forming a single circumscribed mass as in carnivores or monkeys. The ratio SOL/SOM is lower in man than in most primates. While this may be interpreted as evidence for a regression of the SOL, the human SOM has more cells (approximately 11,400) than in any other primate reported, thus reducing the ratio.

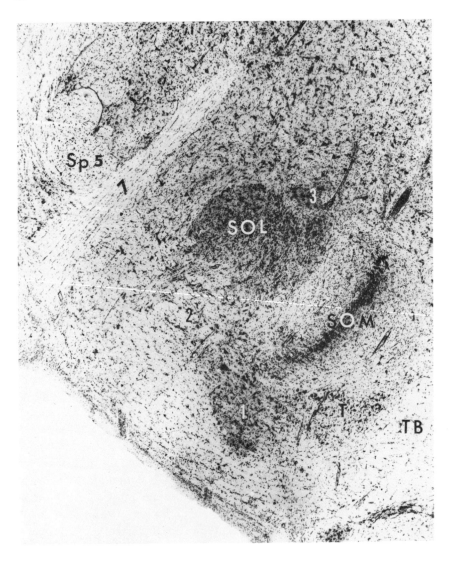

Fig. 5. Photomicrograph of a transverse section of the left superior olivary complex of the rhesus monkey. The medial superior olivary nucleus (SOM) is surrounded medially and laterally by an acellular zone of neuropil. The lateral superior olivary nucleus (SOL) has slight indentations along the dorsal and ventral surfaces. The medial trapezoid nucleus (T) is lateral to the trapezoid body (TB). The medial (1) and lateral (2) preolivary nuclei are diffusely arranged aggregations of cells. The dorsolateral periolivary cell group (3) is the most conspicuous part of the retroolivary group. 7, facial nerve; Sp5, spinal trigeminal tract. Cresyl violet, ×32.

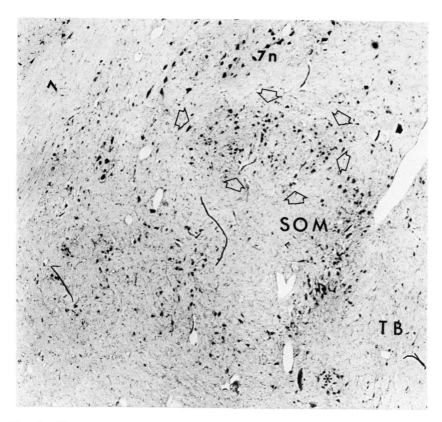

Fig. 6. Photomicrograph of the left superior olivary complex of human. Arrows delimit the lateral superior olivary nucleus. SOM, medial superior olivary nucleus. Asterisk is in cluster of cells possibly forming the medial trapezoid nucleus. Diffusely arranged cells below the medial and lateral superior olivary nuclei constitute the preolivary nuclei. TB, trapezoid body; 7, facial root; 7n, facial nucleus. Cresyl violet, ×32.

2. *Medial Superior Olivary Nucleus.* The SOM is rather constant in shape and the most conspicuous component of the superior olivary complex in all primates (Papez, 1930; Rasmussen, 1946; Stotler, 1953; Moscowitz, 1969). Thus, the term accessory olive, sometimes used for the SOM of nonprimates, is inappropriate. The SOM is a slender, vertically oriented column of cells lying just medial to the SOL. We have counted up to 80 neurons in a single section of the human brain stem.

The SOM in monkey and man may be straight or slightly bowed, with the dorsal tip closer to the midline than the ventral tip. Perikarya commonly are spindle-shaped and emit primary dendrites from both poles. Stotler (1953) showed, in the cat, that these processes pass in medial and lateral directions and receive input from the contralateral and ipsilateral cochlear nuclei respectively.

The ventral tip of the SOM in both the macaque and human contains a number of perikarya which are smaller in size than those present typically at more dorsal locations. The functional significance of these cells is unknown, but they are increased in number in nocturnal primates as noted by Moore and Moore (1971) and may be characteristic of nocturnal mammals generally.

3. *Nucleus of the Trapezoid Body.* The nucleus of the trapezoid body, or medial trapezoid nucleus, is another readily identified segment of the superior olivary complex in the rhesus monkey. The nucleus is located among the fascicles of the trapezoid body ventromedial to the SOM and immediately lateral to the abducens root. Perikarya tend to have smooth round-oval contours in sections stained by the Nissl method. They have finely granular Nissl material and stain darkly. Perikarya of the trapezoid nucleus stand out sharply and are readily differentiated from adjacent cell groups. They are even easier to identify with silver stains. The nucleus has a similar appearance in the brain of the chimpanzee, but we could not identify it with certainty in man (Strominger and Hurwitz, 1976). There are some perikarya ventromedial to the SOM which may represent the nucleus of the trapezoid body, but they are cytoarchitecturally different from neurons of this nucleus in the other species studied. Certainly, the nucleus is at most poorly defined in man. Moore and Moore (1971) also were unsure about its existence in the human. Olszewski and Baxter (1954) labeled the medial trapezoid nucleus and showed some cells similar to those we have seen in the same location; they commented that it is not as well developed in man as in other species.

4. *Preolivary and Periolivary Cell Groups.* In addition to the main nuclei described above, other poorly delimited cell groups are recognized as belonging to the superior olivary complex. Diffusely arranged cells which form a continuum ventral to the SOM and SOL are referred to as the medial preolivary and lateral preolivary nuclei, according to their respective positions with regard to the major segments. Perikarya dorsal to the SOL and SOM constitute the

retroolivary cell group. The lateral part of this group in the macaque consists of a mixture of cells, some of which are larger than those of the SOL. These occupy the area just above the dorsal indentation of the latter, as was illustrated by Ramón y Cajal (1909, p. 813) in the cat, and are also called the dorsolateral periolivary cell group. Perikarya along the dorsomedial aspect of the SOL and above the SOM similarly are called the dorsal periolivary nucleus, which is the medial part of the retroolivary group. Neurons adjacent to the medial side of the SOM, according to their respective positions, are part of the dorsomedial or ventromedial periolivary cell groups.

C. Ventral and Dorsal Nuclei of the Lateral Lemniscus

The nuclei of the lateral lemniscus, located along the course of the fiber bundle bearing the same name, extend from just cephalic to the superior olivary complex in the caudal pons through much of the inferior colliculus (Fig. 7). Two nuclei are distinguished, ventral and dorsal. The ventral nucleus of the lateral lemniscus (VNLL) first appears more caudally than the dorsal nucleus, immediately rostral to the lateral preolivary nucleus. It is a compact aggregation of cells in the ventrolateral part of the tegmentum surrounded ventrally and laterally by fibers of the lateral lemniscus. This bundle forms an angle just lateral to the medial lemniscus prior to assuming a completely vertical orientation at more cephalic levels. The VNLL diminishes in size as the dorsal nucleus of the lateral lemniscus (DNLL) begins and reaches full development. The latter is composed of scattered perikarya, occurring singly and in clusters, located within and separated by fascicles of the lateral lemniscus. This now vertically oriented bundle stretches virtually the entire dorsoventral extent of the tegmentum near the lateral surface. The oral end of the tract and the DNLL underlie the inferior colliculus. The VNLL and the DNLL are cytoarchitecturally distinct, though spatially interconnected by cells bridging fibers of the lateral lemniscus interposed between them where they coexist.

D. Inferior Colliculus

The inferior colliculi are two large nuclear masses which appear as paired rounded protuberances on the posterior surface of the primate brain stem at the level of the caudal midbrain (Fig. 8). More than one

set of terms has been used to describe the various subnuclei of the inferior colliculus. The largest component occupies the central core of the
structure and was called simply the nucleus of the posterior quadri-
geminal tubercle by Ramón y Cajal (1911). This part of the inferior
colliculus constitutes the central nucleus of the inferior colliculus of
contemporary investigators. Ramón y Cajal (1911), who studied several
nonprimates, distinguished external and internuclear cortices as addi-

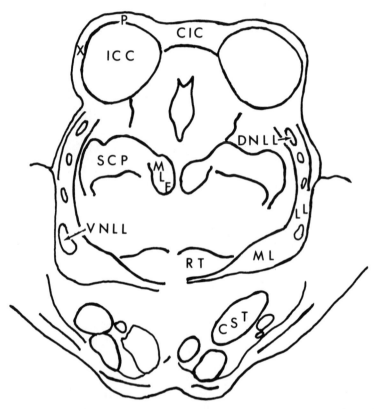

Fig. 7. Projection drawing of a coronal section showing the position of the lateral
lemniscus and its nuclei relative to the inferior colliculus and other structures. The brain
stem is cut obliquely so that the ventral part of the drawing is more caudal than the
dorsal part. CIC, commissure of the inferior colliculus; CST, corticospinal tract;
DNLL, dorsal nucleus of the lateral lemniscus; ICC, central nucleus of the inferior
colliculus; LL, lateral lemniscus; ML, medial lemniscus; MLF, medial longitudinal
fasciculus; P, pericentral nucleus of the inferior colliculus; RT, reticulotegmental
nucleus; SCP, superior cerebellar peduncle; VNLL, ventral nucleus of the lateral
lemniscus; X, external nucleus of the inferior colliculus.

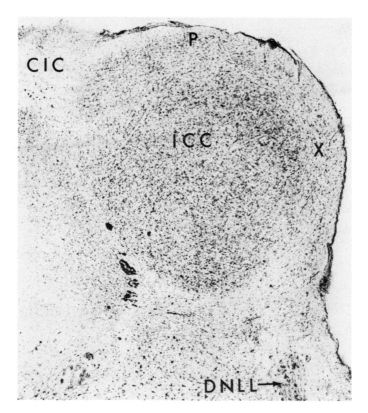

Fig. 8. Photomicrograph of a coronal section through the right inferior colliculus of the rhesus monkey showing the central (ICC), pericentral (P), and external (X) nuclei. The edge of the commissure of the inferior colliculus (CIC) is present, as is the dorsalmost part of the dorsal nucleus of the lateral lemniscus (DNLL) near its anterior end. Cresyl violet, ×20.

tional parts of the inferior colliculus, based on Golgi material. Berman (1968), using Nissl material, also ascribed three parts to the inferior colliculus. According to him, the large central nucleus, composed of densely packed cells, is bordered laterally and rostrally by a band of more loosely arranged cells of similar morphology which constitute the external nucleus of the inferior colliculus. The caudal and dorsal aspects of the central nucleus of the inferior colliculus are covered by even more compactly aggregated cells referred to as the pericentral nucleus. This corresponds to Cajal's internuclear cortex. Examination of the inferior colliculi of the rhesus monkey, chimpanzee, and human reveals a similar organization.

More recently, Geniec and Morest (1971) published a detailed Golgi study of the human inferior colliculus. Several types of neurons with different dendritic properties are present in the central nucleus which occupies the core of the inferior colliculus. The central nucleus is covered by a mainly four-layered cortex which extends from the caudal end of the inferior colliculus over its dorsal aspect to the caudal end of the superior colliculus. The cortex is divided into dorsal and caudal parts. In the caudal cortex, which forms the posterior end of the inferior colliculus, the superficial layers are attenuated. These authors describe a pericollicular tegmentum along the lateral side of the central nucleus and also interposed between it and underlying parts of the tegmentum. This is divided into the intercollicular tegmentum, lateral zone, and cuneiform area. The central nucleus of the inferior colliculus has an encapsulated appearance due to its afferent and efferent myelinated tracts in the pericollicular tegmentum and the superficial cortex.

E. Cell Groups in Proximity to the Brachium of the Inferior Colliculus

The inferior colliculus emits axons which ascend in the brachium of the inferior colliculus. This bundle takes shape along the lateral side of the inferior colliculus and causes a bulge along the lateral surface of the midbrain at levels through the superior colliculus before passing internally to the medial geniculate body, where it terminates. The brachium of the inferior colliculus is mentioned at this time because of perikarya located in geographic proximity to it which undoubtedly participate in the mechanisms of audition. These neurons are located just medial to the brachium of the inferior colliculus at caudal levels; rostrally they intermingle with fibers of the acoustic brachium and end along the ventromedial aspect of the medial geniculate body at its caudal end. Moore and Goldberg (1963, 1966) divide this group of cells in the monkey as well as cat into a more caudal parabrachial region and a rostral interstitial nucleus of the inferior brachium.

F. Medial Geniculate Body

The medial geniculate body, the thalamic component of the main auditory pathways, was considered for several decades to consist of two parts, a lateral densely packed small-celled "parvocellular" or "principal" division (GMp) and a medial "magnocellular" division where the neurons are less compactly arranged and mostly larger in size. The more recent literature suggests that this scheme required modification. Morest (1964, 1965), using Golgi material of the cat, separated the principal division into dorsal and ventral divisions and distinguished a medial division approximating the magnocellular part. He further noted that the ventral division consists of a laminated ventral nucleus (not apparent with Nissl sections) divided into anterolateral and ventromedial areas.

Burton and Jones (1976), using Nissl sections of the squirrel and rhesus monkeys, also separated the GMp into three parts, designated posterodorsal, anterodorsal, and ventral divisions; the term "magnocellular division" was retained to describe the large-celled part of the medial geniculate. Following their terminology, the posterodorsal division occupies the entire caudal pole of the medial geniculate body. The anterodorsal division of the GMp extends through the anterior two-thirds of the nucleus; its caudal end overlies the rostral end of the posterodorsal division (Fig. 9). The cells of the anterodorsal division are said to be somewhat larger than those of the posterodorsal division, but this difference is slight and the exact transition between these parts of the principal division is not readily defined. The ventral division is situated most ventrally in the GMp and has a rostrocaudal range of slightly more than the middle third of the medial geniculate body. A hint of a laminar organization described as rows, spirals, or bands is seen in optimal Nissl material, but this often is not obvious enough to be a distinguishing feature. However, the perikarya stain slightly more intensely than those of the anterodorsal and posterodorsal divisions and are more tightly packed. The magnocellular division of the medial geniculate is located along the medial side of that structure throughout roughly its anterior half. The perikarya are more loosely arranged and mainly larger than those of the GMp. Although there are difficulties in differentiating the precise boundaries of the different parts, especially of the GMp, this organization is useful in that it reflects their differing afferent and efferent connections, and hence functional properties.

G. Auditory Cortex

1. Identification of the Primary Auditory Area in Primates. The general position of the cortical receptive fields for audition have been

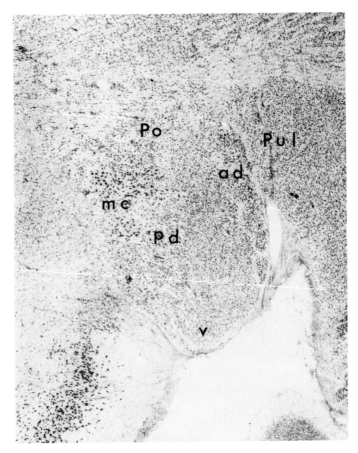

Fig. 9.   Photomicrograph of a coronal section through the right medial geniculate body of the rhesus monkey showing its constituents, including the ventral (v), posterodorsal (pd), and anterodorsal (ad) components of the principal division, and the magnocellular division (mc). Po, posterior group of thalamus; Pul, inferior nucleus of pulvinar. Cresyl violet, ×20.

known for about a century—since the publications of Ferrier (1876, 1890), who observed pricking up of the opposite ear, and head and eye turning as if to sounds, after electrical stimulation of posterior portions of the lateral surface of the superior temporal gyrus in the monkey and part of the ectosylvian gyrus in the cat, dog, and jackal. Cauterization of this region bilaterally in a monkey produced inattention to auditory stimuli. The descriptions and illustrations do not indicate whether cortex buried within the lateral fissure, now known to be the site of the primary auditory cortex, also was cauterized. Ferrier inferred that the superior temporal gyrus also is the center of hearing in man.

Poliak (1932), employing the Marchi method to trace anterograde degeneration after lesions of the medial geniculate in monkeys, determined that the auditory radiations terminate throughout much of the submerged superior surface of the superior temporal gyrus, where they are most concentrated caudally, as well as to a lesser extent on the exposed lateral surface. The superior surface of the superior temporal gyrus, buried within the lower bank of the lateral (Sylvian) fissure, is called the superior (supra)temporal plane. Le Gros Clark (1936), using the retrograde cell change method, restricted the auditory cortex to the small posterior part of Brodmann's (1909) area 22 in the supratemporal plane of the macaque. Walker (1937) correlated experimental observations of retrograde cell changes in the monkey with a study of the cortical cytoarchitecture. He reasoned that the auditory projection area would have a distinct cytoarchitecture similar to the koniocortex already demonstrated for the somatosensory and visual areas. Thus, he determined the limits of the koniocortex, found that small lesions within this area produced degeneration in the medial geniculate, and accurately delimited the primary auditory cortex to a small area within the posterior half of the superior temporal plane.

Results of several electrophysiological studies have shown that there is a topographic representation of the cochlea, or tonotopic organization, toward the caudal end of the superior temporal plane of the macaque (Licklider and Kryter, 1942; Bailey *et al.*, 1943; Walzl and Woolsey, 1943; Woolsey and Walzl, 1944; Walzl, 1947; Kennedy, 1955; Merzenich and Brugge, 1973), owl monkey (Imig *et al.*, 1977), and chimpanzee (Bailey *et al.*, 1943; Woolsey, 1972). High frequencies are represented caudomedially and low frequencies rostrolaterally in the primary auditory cortex (Fig. 10). The spatial layout reflects the obliqueness of this part of the superior temporal plane. A slight protuberance is present here.

Other investigators have confirmed electrophysiologically that the auditory areas are similarly located in the human temporal lobe (Penfield and Perot, 1963; Celesia and Puletti, 1969). The primary auditory cortex occupies parts of two obliquely directed elevations upon the superior temporal plane—the anterior and posterior transverse temporal gyri (Heschl's gyri), which lie on either side of the transverse supratemporal sulcus. Heschl's gyri are the site of areas 41 and 42 of

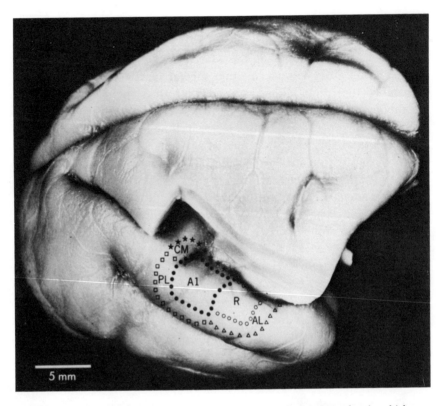

Fig. 10.   Photograph of the right cerebral hemisphere of an owl monkey in which part of the frontoparietal operculum has been removed to expose the superior temporal plane. Locations of five auditory fields determined cytoarchitectonically and electrophysiologically are shown. The first auditory field (A1) and the rostral field (R) in this species form a central core of auditory cortex. This is surrounded by a belt of cortical fields designated caudomedial (CM), posterolateral (PL), and anterolateral (AL) in which units generally are less responsive to acoustic stimuli and where the frequency organization is more complex. (From Imig et al., 1977; courtesy of Wistar Institute Press.)

Brodmann (1909), which also extend onto the superior temporal gyrus (Fig. 11). They are surrounded by areas 22 and 52, which are partially situated on the supratemporal plane. The primary auditory cortex includes parts of areas 41 and 42. According to Celesia and Puletti (1969), there is some variability in the number of transverse temporal gyri, but two are usual.

    2. *The Primary Auditory Cortex in Cat.*   Rose (1949) [as had Bremer and Dow (1939)] identified in the cat a cortical region similar

to that described by Walker. He also noted that the characterization of the koniocortex must be broadened to include the primary auditory cortex under this classification. In the primary auditory area, which he termed AI, perikarya generally are small and densely packed throughout layers II–IV, thereby blurring the lamination. The perikarya have a small range in size through all layers. Layers V and VI are readily distinguished because of a relatively sparse cellularity of the former. Rose added that his observations generally are applicable to descriptions of this field in man (Economo and Koskinas, 1925). This description of AI can be applied to recent cytoarchitectural analyses of the auditory cortex in the macaque (Merzenich and Brugge, 1973).

3. *Other Cortical Auditory Areas in Cat.* In addition to the central field, AI, Rose considered that the auditory region of the cat also included a surrounding peripheral belt of cortex which was transitional in form. The granular and supragranular layers resembled AI in many respects; the infragranular layers mainly were characteristic of adjoining cortical fields. The heterogeneous peripheral belt was divided into three fields: auditory area II (AII), below the central field and above the tip of the pseudosylvian sulcus; the posterior ectosylvian area (Ep),

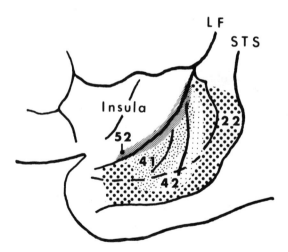

Fig. 11.   Schematic drawing of the human cerebral cortex showing the region of the lateral fissure, which is opened to illustrate the transverse temporal gyri (largely occupied by areas 41 and 42) and the adjacent insula. The superior temporal gyrus extends between the lateral fissure (LF) and the superior temporal sulcus (STS) and is located on the lateral surface of the brain. The top of the temporal lobe is toward the left. (Slightly modified from Brodmann, 1909.)

behind AI and occupying much of the posterior ectosylvian gyrus; and the suprasylvian fringe area, located along the dorsal bank of the suprasylvian sulcus, extending to the fundus where it borders AI. At that time there was no evidence to suggest a functional role in auditory mechanisms for the suprasylvian fringe area, so the term "auditory belt" at first was used to designate AII and Ep. Subsequent anatomical studies using the retrograde cell change method together with behavioral and electrophysiological investigations led to a redelineation of auditory cortex in the cat which incorporated additional regions including the insular-temporal area and a region designated auditory area III, anterior to the ventral end of the anterior ectosylvian sulcus [for cortical map, see Woolsey (1960)]. Details of the organization of the thalamocortical part of the auditory system are provided in a recent review by Neff et al. (1975).

4. *Other Cortical Auditory Areas in the Monkey.* Compared to the cat, fewer experiments have explored the thalamocortical portion of the primate auditory system. This is attributable largely to the relative inaccessibility of the auditory cortex in primates, where it is buried within the depths of the lateral fissure. There also is a lack of conspicuous sulci, which in the cat while not necessarily limiting sulci nevertheless are useful guides for locating the various auditory subdivisions. Also, cats were used preferentially in numerous behavioral experiments for a variety of reasons. Over the last several years a considerable amount of work has been published on the thalamocortical as well as other levels of the primate auditory system.

Merzenich and Brugge (1973) in a combined cytoarchitectural and electrophysiological study extended Rose's (1949) observations to the cortex of the macaque. The auditory type of koniocortex characteristic of AI was localized in the same area within the posterior part of the superior temporal plane delimited earlier by Walker (1937).

A complete frequency representation was found in AI in agreement with other studies, as has been mentioned earlier—with high frequencies (base of cochlea) represented rostrolaterally and low frequencies (apex) caudomedially. This sequence is the reverse of the topographic organization in the cat and is attributed to a rotation of the temporal lobe about the insula that occurs with development of the primate cerebral hemispheres (Woolsey, 1972). This alters the spatial relationships of the other auditory areas with respect to each other and to AI. Thus, based on a reversal of the tonotopicity relative to AI, AII has been located medial to the primary auditory area and extending onto the superior bank of the lateral fissure in the parietal operculum (Woolsey and Fairman, 1946; Walzl, 1947; Woolsey, 1972). According to Woolsey, the homologue of the posterior ectosylvian field is situated rostral to AI rather than caudal to it as in the cat, and the suprasylvian fringe area is caudal to AI instead of rostral.

Sanides (1972) divided primary auditory cortex of the macaque into two cyto- and myeloarchitectonically distinct fields of koniocortex which are in parallel, with one medial to the other. He noted that this is equivalent to the organization of auditory koniocortex in man. While Merzenich and Brugge (1973) described a single cytoarchitectural field in the macaque, Imig et al. (1977) found that the auditory koniocortex of the owl monkey is not uniform everywhere. Nonetheless, they agree that following the criterion of its frequency organization, AI forms a single field. Of interest was the finding that the primary auditory cortex of the owl monkey extends onto the superior temporal gyrus. Brodmann (1909) showed area 41 and 42 to an even greater extent, passing out onto the surface of the first temporal convolution.

Sanides (1972) described a belt of architectonically transitional cortex surrounding AI which was separated into several fields. Merzenich and Brugge (1973) and Imig et al. (1977) also found in the rhesus and owl monkeys respectively several cytoarchitecturally distinct regions of transitional cortex and explored some of their physiological properties (see Fig. 10). The terminology used to designate the various subdivisions of auditory cortex thus defined and their domains is not constant. At the present time it is clear that some of the fields are tonotopically organized in the same manner as AI and that the response characteristics to sound of other fields are more complicated.

Studies in man in which click-evoked responses have been recorded from part of the lateral surface of the superior temporal gyrus and the frontal and parietal operculi confirm the presence of auditory fields outside of the primary areas (Celesia, 1976).

III. The Course and Distribution of Primary Auditory Fibers

The topographic relationships between different portions of the auditory receptor organ and the cochlear nuclei have been analyzed in the squirrel monkey by Moscowitz and Liu (1972), who determined that each turn of the cochlea projects to all three major subdivisions of the cochlear complex. The central axons of fibers in the cochlear root bifurcate to form ascending and descending branches. Fibers in the ascending branch supply the anteroventral cochlear nucleus, while those

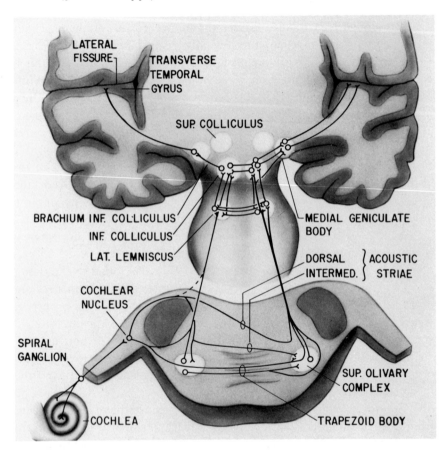

Fig. 12. Schematic drawing presenting a simplified representation of the ascending auditory pathways starting from one cochlea, based on studies in the rhesus monkey and chimpanzee. The cochlear nucleus of this drawing represents all three subdivisions of the cochlear complex whose individual efferent connections to the superior olivary complex are shown in Fig. 13. Similarly the lateral lemniscus in this diagram refers to both the ventral and dorsal nuclei of the lateral lemniscus. Fibers between the inferior colliculus and medial geniculate body are located in the brachium of the inferior colliculus. The geniculocortical radiations pass through the sublenticular portion of the posterior limb of the internal capsule. The commissures of the lateral lemniscus and inferior colliculus also are not labeled.

in the descending branch pass into the posteroventral and dorsal cochlear nuclei. Basal to apical turns of the spiral ganglion project in a dorsomedial to ventrolateral sequence in each subdivision.

Fibers in the ascending branch from base to apex of the cochlea also are arranged in a caudomedial to rostrolateral direction. The large spherical cells receive input only from the apical and to a lesser extent middle turns of the cochlea in this species. The small spherical cells and globular cells are supplied by all turns of the spiral ganglion. Given that the base of the cochlea is where high frequencies are mediated, and that low frequencies activate hair cells nearer the apex of the cochlea, these findings suggest that the large spherical cells are involved in mechanisms of hearing only toward the low end of the frequency spectrum. This conforms to the tonotopic organization of the Av (Rose *et al.*, 1959, 1960). While we have not found separate populations of small and large spherical cells in the rhesus monkey and human, a similar topographic relationship with the cochlea and tonotopic organization of second-order neurons doubtless exists.

Fibers in the descending branch of the cochlear root are said to terminate in association with multipolar and octopus cells in the Pv as well as globular cells located in orodorsal parts of the Pv in this species. The multipolar neurons are supplied by fibers from all turns of the spiral ganglion, and the octopus cells are supplied mainly from the apical turn. Primary fibers from throughout the spiral ganglion enter the DCN and terminate in the central and pyramidal layers. No primary fibers are known to pass beyond the level of the cochlear nuclei, as illustrated in Fig. 12, which is a simplified diagram of the entire ascending auditory pathways.

IV. Ascending Fiber Systems in the Central Nervous System

A. Fibers Arising from the Cochlear Nuclei

1. Projections to the Superior Olivary Complex.   The course and distribution of second-order auditory fibers emanating from the three major subdivisions of the cochlear nuclei were determined in the rhesus monkey (Strominger and Strominger, 1971; Strominger, 1973). Stereotactically placed lesions were produced in the anteroventral cochlear nucleus, the dorsal cochlear nucleus, and in the posteroventral

nucleus in combination with each of the other subdivisions; resulting degeneration was studied using the Nauta–Gygax (1954) and
Fink–Heimer (1967) techniques for tracing anterograde degeneration.
The projections of the cochlear nuclei upon the individual segments of
the superior olivary complex and their contribution to the three auditory
decussations in the caudal pons are illustrated in Fig. 13. The DCN
gives rise to fibers which arch around the superior surface of the restiform body to pass mesad into the region of the vestibular complex. This
fascicle, comprising the dorsal acoustic stria of Monakow, courses in a
medioventral direction to cross the midline in a relatively dorsal position
within the tegmentum, though its fibers are more diffusely organized
than illustrated. Its fibers approach the contralateral superior olivary
complex from above. In the monkey it appeared as though a few fibers
terminated in the lateral superior olivary nucleus, but studies in a chimpanzee with extensive damage involving all three subdivisions of the
cochlear nuclei failed to confirm this observation (Strominger *et al.*,
1977). It seems likely that fibers in the dorsal acoustic stria entirely
bypass the superior olivary complex and ascend directly to more
cephalic levels of the auditory pathway.

Fibers emerging from the Pv traverse the dorsal subdivision and
coalesce with axons from the latter to pass around the restiform body
and enter the tegmentum. Fibers taking origin within the Pv form the
intermediate acoustic stria of Held. They turn downward in the ipsilateral tegmentum medial to the restiform body, and approach the
dorsal aspect of the superior olivary complex. These fibers, relatively
few in number, are distributed to retroolivary and preolivary cell groups
as well as to the SOL. The intermediate acoustic stria continues across
the midline just above the trapezoid body, and its fibers are distributed
to retroolivary and preolivary groups as on the ipsilateral side. Observations in the chimpanzee suggest that there probably are no terminations
of this fascicle in the contralateral SOL as reported earlier in the
monkey. Thus, the Pv projects mainly to periolivary and preolivary cell
groups. It has been known for some time, since the elegant experiments
by Rasmussen (1946, 1960, 1964) in the cat and other species, that
some of these nuclei give rise to fibers which comprise the olivocochlear
bundle and terminate directly on hair cells to affect the afferent input
(Galambos, 1956; Kimura and Wersäll, 1962; Spoendlin and Gacek,
1963; Smith and Rasmussen, 1965).

By far the largest number of second-order auditory fibers arise

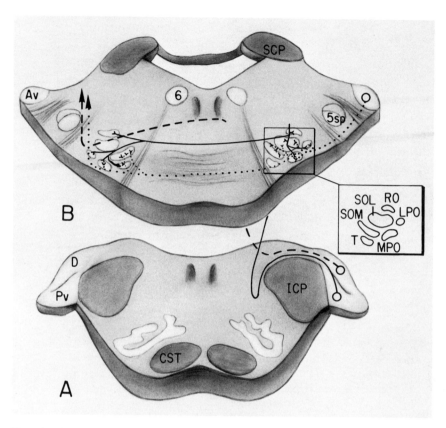

Fig. 13. Semischematic drawings show the projections of the dorsal, posteroventral, and anteroventral cochlear nuclei upon the various subnuclei of the superior olivary complex as elucidated in the rhesus monkey. The dorsal cochlear nucleus (DCN) gives rise to axons which form the dorsal acoustic stria (dashed line). This fascicle mainly or entirely bypasses the superior olivary complex and ascends to more cephalic levels, as shown by the arrowhead, in the contralateral lateral lemniscus. The posteroventral cochlear nucleus (Pv) gives rise to axons which form the intermediate acoustic stria (solid line). These fibers are distributed bilaterally to the retroolivary (RO) and preolivary [lateral (LPO) and medial (MPO)] cell groups, to the ipsilateral lateral superior olive (SOL) and to the contralateral nucleus of the trapezoid body (T). The anteroventral cochlear nucleus (Av) gives rise to axons which cross the vestibular and facial roots to enter the trapezoid body (dotted line). These fibers are distributed to the ipsilateral lateral superior olive, contralateral nucleus of the trapezoid body, and bilaterally to the preolivary and medial superior olivary nuclei. Fibers project to the lateral and medial sides of the ipsilateral and contralateral medial superior olivary nuclei respectively. Not shown are fibers which ascend in the ipsilateral lateral lemniscus. CST, corticospinal tract; ICP, inferior cerebellar peduncle; SCP, superior cerebellar peduncle; 5SP, spinal trigeminal tract and nucleus; 6, abducens nucleus.

from the Av and pass mesad beneath the spinal trigeminal tract and nucleus to enter and form the lateral part of the trapezoid body. This bundle, also referred to as the ventral acoustic stria, decussates in the ventral part of the tegmentum and contains more fibers than the dorsal and intermediate acoustic striae combined, as noted by Barnes *et al.* (1943). The trapezoid body, in complete contrast to the other acoustic striae, is clearly visible in normal Weigert preparations. It is most conspicuous at medial locations between the superior olivary nuclei of the two sides. Here, it contains transversely oriented auditory fibers, taking origin both from the anteroventral cochlear nuclei and the superior olivary complex bilaterally, which intermingle with the longitudinally coursing fibers of the medial lemniscus. Fibers from the Av are distributed profusely to the ipsilateral SOL and to laterally and medially oriented dendrites of the ipsilateral and contralateral medial superior olives respectively. Some fibers appear to end upon soma of the SOM. There also are bilateral projections to the lateral and medial preolivary nuclei and projections to the contralateral nucleus of the trapezoid body.

Data in the monkey indicate the presence of a topographic projection from the Av to the SOM with dorsal parts of the Av sending fibers to the ventral part of the latter. This conforms to the tonotopic organization of these subnuclei elucidated in the cat and dog; high frequencies are represented in the dorsal Av and in what corresponds to the ventral tip of the SOM (Rose *et al.*, 1959, 1960; Goldberg and Brown, 1968).

2. *Second-Order Projections to the Nuclei of the Lateral Lemniscus and Inferior Colliculus.* Axons which take origin from the dorsal and anteroventral cochlear nuclei, ascend in part beyond the level of the superior olivary complex. These fibers enter the contralateral lateral lemniscus, where they are distributed mainly to the ventral nucleus, though some go to the dorsal nucleus of the lateral lemniscus. A large number continue through the lateral lemniscus and terminate within the central nucleus of the inferior colliculus. It is uncertain from our material whether some fibers also come from the posteroventral cochlear nucleus, but evidence in the cat indicates that they do (see Fig. 14).

Uncrossed fibers from the Av project abundantly upon perikarya at the caudal pole of the VNLL, but few terminate in rostral parts of either the VNLL or the DNLL. Some fibers reach the ipsilateral central nucleus of the inferior colliculus. The DCN and Pv emit few fibers that go to the ipsilateral nuclei of the lateral lemniscus, though scattered

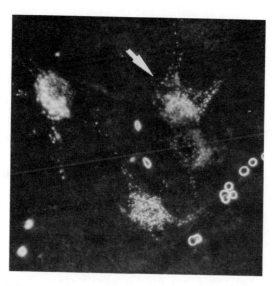

Fig. 14. Dark-field photomicrograph showing retrograde labeling of octopus cell (arrow) and other neurons in Pv of cat following injection of horseradish peroxidase into the central nucleus of the inferior colliculus. ×750. (Courtesy of Drs. Judy Brunso-Bechtold and Glenn Thompson.)

uncrossed degeneration is seen in the central nucleus of the inferior colliculus after lesions restricted to the DCN or involving it together with the Pv.

3. *The Question of Direct Projections from the Cochlear Nuclei to the Thalamus.* Of interest is the question whether any second-order auditory fibers pass directly to thalamic levels. The auditory pathway is considered different from other sensory systems in having an additional mandatory relay prior to the thalamus. Ramón y Cajal (1909) held the view that some fibers originating in the cochlear nuclei ascend directly to the medial geniculate body. Most subsequent investigators using techniques for studying anterograde degeneration have not confirmed this connection, including Barnes *et al.* (1943) in the monkey. The results of studies in nonprimates led to the conclusion that this link does not exist. A few degenerating fibers were noted in the contralateral magnocellular division of the medial geniculate body of the macaque following lesions of the cochlear nuclei in experiments done in our laboratory, but they were inconstant and quantitatively negligible. Recently, a fair amount of unequivocal degeneration was traced through the contralateral bra-

chium of the inferior colliculus into both the ventral nucleus of the principal division of the medial geniculate body and the magnocellular division after aspiration of the cochlear nuclei in a chimpanzee (Strominger *et al.*, 1977). These findings suggest the establishment of a phylogenetic advance in the auditory pathway of the great ape. It should be noted, as will be discussed later, that projections to the medial geniculate body were not to the dorsal nucleus of the principal division.

B. Efferent Connections of the Superior Olivary Complex

Results of studies of the ascending connections of the superior olivary complex are difficult to evaluate. Techniques whereby lesions are produced either in the complex as a whole or in individual segments and anterograde degeneration is traced using any of several methods are limited in reliability because fibers of passage interrupted by an electrode track or lesion are also stained. Individual subnuclei of the superior olivary complex are traversed by axons arising from other segments of the complex on the same and opposite sides, as well as by fibers emanating from the cochlear nuclei on both sides. The recently developed autoradiographic methods for studying anterograde transport of proteins eliminate this problem. With the use of horseradish peroxidase to label cells in a retrograde direction, a clearer picture of the efferent connections of the superior olivary complex should emerge over the next several years.

At the present time, based on studies in the cat (Rasmussen, 1946, 1964; Stotler, 1953; Van Noort, 1969; Brunso-Bechtold and Thompson, 1976), rabbit (Borg, 1973), and kangaroo rat (Browner and Webster, 1975), one can conclude with certainty that the lateral superior olivary nucleus projects bilaterally to the central nucleus of the inferior colliculus and probably to the dorsal nucleus of the lateral lemniscus. The medial superior olivary nucleus gives rise to uncrossed fibers which enter the lateral lemniscus and go to the central nucleus of the inferior colliculus. That the ventral as well as dorsal nuclei of the lateral lemniscus receive projections from both the SOL and SOM seems probable but has not been conclusively demonstrated. Recent studies with horseradish peroxidase indicate that the inferior colliculus receives some fibers from the periolivary region, but precise details are lacking in this preliminary report (Brunso-Bechtold and Thompson, 1976).

Although Barnes *et al.* (1943) concluded that in the monkey some fibers from the superior olivary complex reach the medial geniculate body, it seems likely that in their study the lesion interrupted fibers of spinal origin.

C. Projections of the Nuclei of the Lateral Lemniscus

The efferent connections of the VNLL have not been firmly established. Some fibers originating here apparently terminate at least in the ipsilateral DNLL and in the central nucleus of the inferior colliculus. The latter may be an important link in the uncrossed auditory pathways, since, as has been mentioned earlier, the caudal pole of the VNLL receives strong projections from the ipsilateral Av.

The DNLL gives rise to fibers which project massively to the ipsilateral central nucleus of the inferior colliculus (Goldberg and Moore, 1967). A smaller fascicle crosses the midline in the commissure of the lateral lemniscus (commissure of Probst) to partially terminate in the opposite DNLL and in part to ascend to the central nucleus of the inferior colliculus. It should be noted that the commissure of the lateral lemniscus is not visible in myelin preparations of normal material.

D. Projections of the Inferior Colliculus

The central nucleus is the principal output nucleus of the inferior colliculus. Some fibers emerging from it are distributed to the external nucleus. The largest number of ascending fibers pass into the ipsilateral brachium of the inferior colliculus. They are in part distributed throughout its parabrachial and interstitial nuclei but mainly continue to the medial geniculate body, where they go to the rostral four-fifths of the principal division and to the magnocellular division (Moore and Goldberg, 1966). Another smaller fascicle reaches the contralateral brachium of the inferior colliculus via the commissure of the inferior colliculus and has a similar thalamic distribution as the uncrossed component; en route, fibers are given off to the central nucleus of the inferior colliculus, to the pericentral and external nuclei, and to the parabrachial and interstitial nuclei of the acoustic brachium.

E. Efferent Connections of the Parabrachial and Interstitial Nuclei of the Brachium of the Inferior Colliculus

As indicated, both the parabrachial region and interstitial nucleus of the brachium of the inferior colliculus receive afferent input from the central nucleus of the inferior colliculus. According to Morest (1965), who made an extensive study of fiber systems ascending in the lateral part of the midbrain tegmentum in the cat, lesions involving the brachium of the inferior colliculus and the region just medial to it produce degeneration in what he defines as the deep part of the dorsal nucleus of the medial geniculate body. This thalamic area does not contain preterminal degeneration after lesions of the inferior colliculus.

The efferent connections of the interstitial nucleus of the brachium of the inferior colliculus are uncertain at the present time. If it is a rostral continuation of the parabrachial region, as suggested by some investigators, it may emit similar efferents to the medial geniculate.

F. Geniculocortical Projections

The auditory radiations from the medial geniculate body traverse the sublenticular portion of the posterior limb of the internal capsule before reaching the region of the supratemporal plane. The precise manner in which parts of the medial geniculate project to subdivisions of auditory cortex has been determined by a combination of methods. The retrograde cell change method was applied very successfully, as will be described below, in initially establishing details of the thalamocortical portion of the cat auditory system. In the monkey, recent studies employing autoradiographic tracing techniques have been most useful.

1. Retrograde Degeneration in the Medial Geniculate Body of the Cat. Simultaneous with Rose's (1949) cytoarchitectural study showing that auditory cortex is constituted of more than one distinct region, Rose and Woolsey (1949) reported that small lesions in different parts of AI produce focal degeneration within the principal division of the medial geniculate body in an orderly manner. Lesions in rostral AI caused cell loss in the rostral GMp and lesions in caudal AI caused cell loss near the middle of the GMp. The posterior third, approximately, of the GMp was preserved after ablations of almost all of AI. The degenerated region corresponds to the ventral division of the GMp. Rose and

Woolsey used the term "essential projections" to denote the efferent connections from the GMp to AI. In this type of projection, a small lesion causes definite retrograde degeneration so that a clear connection is established between two loci. In contrast, they were unable to demonstrate any thalamic projections to AII or Ep with small ablations limited to these areas of cortex. Later, they showed that the GMp does emit axons which go to cortical areas outside AI (Rose and Woolsey, 1958). The term "sustaining projection" was introduced to describe a situation where ablation of two separate areas individually causes no thalamic degeneration, but ablation of both produces profound cellular alterations. Thus, they showed that the GMp sends sustaining projections to AII and Ep and surmised that it possibly sends such projections to both the insular and temporal cortices as well. The most likely explanation of the phenomenon of sustaining projections was based upon the assumption that if a cell has two or more axon collaterals, preservation of one of them, as might occur after a small cortical lesion, would suffice to maintain its structural integrity. A projection from the caudal pole of the GMp to the insular and temporal areas was demonstrated by Diamond *et al.* (1958).

The posterior group of thalamic nuclei also projects to the auditory cortex. The magnocellular division of the medial geniculate exhibits degenerative changes after larger cortical ablations and is considered to emit sustaining projections to AI, AII, Ep, and the insular-temporal cortex. Other parts of the posterior group may be affected by extensive lesions of the auditory cortex.

Anterograde degeneration methods have also been employed to elucidate the organization of the projections from the thalamus to different parts of auditory cortex (Heath and Jones, 1971; Sousa-Pinto, 1973).

2. Studies in the Monkey. While early studies using the retrograde cell change method established the projection from the rostral part of the principal division of the medial geniculate body to the primary auditory cortex in the monkey, the relationships between the thalamus and the cortex have not been elaborated with this technique in as complete detail as in the cat. Akert *et al.* (1959) showed that ablations of the supratemporal plane anterior to the primary auditory cortex produce cell loss at the caudal pole of the GMp. Recent experiments tracing anterograde transport of labeled protein are in essential agreement (Burton and Jones, 1976).

They show that the ventral division of the GMp sends fibers to the primary auditory cortex and suggest that subpopulations within the posterodorsal component of the GMp have distinct cortical projection fields in areas anterior and medial to AI. Mesulam and Pandya (1973), using silver impregnation techniques, concluded that the caudal third of the GMp projects to the superior temporal plane anterior to the primary auditory cortex as well as to the superior temporal gyrus. Burton and Jones (1976) found label in the superior temporal gyrus only after injections involving the anterodorsal component of the GMp, but they were unable to specify the exact origin of this projection. Results of behavioral studies show that the supratemporal plane anterior to AI and the superior temporal gyrus are important for some kinds of auditory discrimination (Neff, 1961; Dewson *et al.*, 1970; Wegener, 1976; Strominger *et al.*, 1978). According to Burton and Jones (1976), the magnocellular division of the medial geniculate body projects diffusely to layer I of all auditory fields. Parts of the posterior group of nuclei adjacent to the anterodorsal division of the GMp appear to send fibers to the auditory cortex posterior to AI.

V. Other Connections

The preceding sections have been concerned with the nuclear complexes and ascending fiber connections of the auditory pathway, with particular emphasis on primates. Without going into details, it should be mentioned that the auditory system is constituted of other important components. A descending pathway extends from the cerebral cortex to the hair cells of the cochlea. The olivocochlear bundle mentioned earlier, the last part of this system, has been studied extensively since its initial description in the cat (Rasmussen, 1946) and has been shown to exist in man (Gacek, 1961). Through this pathway the central part of the auditory system can affect its afferent input. There also are connections to the motor trigeminal and facial nuclei which mediate the efferent limb of the middle ear reflex, and possible connections to the superior colliculus, cerebellum, and other structures. Thus, auditory stimuli activate complicated and widespread neural pathways.

Acknowledgments.   This manuscript was written during a sabbatical in the Department of Anatomy and Neurobiology, Washington

University, St. Louis. The many courtesies extended by Dr. W. M. Cowan and the Department are greatly appreciated.

VI. References

Akert, K., Woolsey, C. N., Diamond, I. T., and Neff, W. D. 1959. The cortical projection area of the posterior pole of the medial geniculate body in *Macaca mulatta*, *Anat. Rec. 134*:242.

Bacsik, R. D., and Strominger, N. L. 1973. The cytoarchitecture of the human anteroventral cochlear nucleus. *J. Comp. Neurol. 147*:281–290.

Bailey, P., Bonin, G. v., Garol, H. W., and McCulloch, W. S. 1943. Functional organization of temporal lobe of monkey (*Macaca mulatta*) and chimpanzee (*Pan satyrus*). *J. Neurophysiol. 6*:121–128.

Barnes, W. T., Magoun, H. W., and Ranson, S. W. 1943. The ascending auditory pathway in the brain stem of the monkey. *J. Comp. Neurol. 79*:129–152.

Berman, A. L. 1968. *The brain stem of the cat. A cytoarchitectonic atlas with stereotaxic coordinates*. University of Wisconsin, Madison. 175 pp.

Borg, E. 1973. A neuroanatomical study of the brain stem auditory system of the rabbit. Part I. Ascending connections. *Acta Morphol. Neerl. Scand. 11*:31–48.

Brawer, J. R., Morest, D. K., and Kane, E. C. 1974. The neuronal architecture of the cochlear nucleus of the cat. *J. Comp. Neurol. 155*:251–300.

Bremer, F., and Dow, R. S. 1939. The acoustic area of the cerebral cortex in the cat: A combined oscillographic and cytoarchitectonic study. *J. Neurophysiol. 2*:308–318.

Brodmann, K. 1909. *Vergleichende Lokalisationslehre der Grosshirnrinde*. J. A. Barth, Leipzig. 324 pp.

Browner, R. H., and Webster, D. B. 1975. Projections of the trapezoid body and the superior olivary complex of the kangaroo rat (*Dipodomys merriami*). *Brain Behav. Evol. 11*:322–354.

Brunso-Bechtold, J. K., and Thompson, G. C. 1976. Auditory hindbrain projections to the inferior colliculus as demonstrated by horseradish peroxidase in the cat. *Anat. Rec. 184*:365.

Burton, H., and Jones, E. G. 1976. The posterior thalamic region and its cortical projection in New World and Old World monkeys. *J. Comp. Neurol. 168*:249–302.

Celesia, G. G. 1976. Organization of auditory cortical areas in man. *Brain 99*:403–414.

Celesia, G. G., and Puletti, F. 1969. Auditory cortical areas of man. *Neurology 19*:211–220.

Clark, W. E. Le Gros 1936. The thalamic connections of the temporal lobe of the brain in the monkey. *J. Anat. 70*:447–464.

Dewson, J. H., III, Cowey, A., and Weiskrantz, L. 1970. Disruptions of auditory sequence discrimination by unilateral and bilateral cortical ablations of superior temporal gyrus in the monkey. *Exp. Neurol. 28*:529–548.

Diamond, I. T., Chow, K. L., and Neff, W. D. 1958. Degeneration of caudal medial geniculate body following cortical lesion ventral to auditory area II in cat. *J. Comp. Neurol. 109*:349–362.

Economo, C. v., and Koskinas, G. N. 1925. *Die Cytoarchitektonik der Hirnrinde der erwachsenen Menschen.* J. Springer, Vienna. 810 pp.

Ferrier, D. 1876. *The Functions of the Brain.* Smith, Elder, London. 323 pp.

Ferrier, D. 1890. The Croonian lectures on cerebral localization. Lecture IV—The auditory centre. *Br. Med. J. 1* (for 1890):1473–1479.

Fink, R. P., and Heimer, L. 1967. Two methods for selective impregnation of degenerating axons and their synaptic endings in the central nervous system. *Brain Res. 4:*369–374.

Gacek, R. R. 1961. The efferent cochlear bundle in man. *Arch. Otolaryngol. 74:*690–694.

Galambos, R. 1956. Suppression of auditory nerve activity by stimulation of efferent fibers to cochlea. *J. Neurophysiol. 19:*424–437.

Geniec, P., and Morest, D. K. 1971. The neuronal architecture of the human posterior colliculus. A study with the Golgi method. *Acta. Oto-Laryngol. Suppl. 295:*1–33.

Goldberg, J. M., and Brown, P. B. 1968. Functional organization of the dog superior olivary complex: An anatomical and electrophysiological study. *J. Neurophysiol. 31:*649–656.

Goldberg, J. M., and Moore, R. Y. 1967. Ascending projections of the lateral lemniscus in the cat and monkey. *J. Comp. Neurol. 129:*143–156.

Heath, C. J., and Jones, E. G. 1971. An experimental study of ascending connections from the posterior group of thalamic nuclei in the cat. *J. Comp. Neurol. 141:*397–426.

Imig, T. J., Ruggero, M. A., Kitzes, L. M., Javel, E., and Brugge, J. F. 1977. Organization of auditory cortex in the owl monkey (*Aotus trivirgatus*). *J. Comp. Neurol. 171:*111–128.

Kennedy, T. T. 1955. An electrophysiological study of the auditory projection areas of the cortex in monkey (*Macaca mulatta*). Doctoral Dissertation, University of Chicago.

Kimura, R., and Wersäll, J. 1962. Termination of the olivocochlear bundle in relation to the outer hair cells of the organ of Corti in guinea pig. *Acta. Oto-Laryngol. 55:*11–32.

Le Gros Clark, see Clark.

Licklider, J. C. R., and Kryter, K. D. 1942. Frequently localization in the auditory cortex of the monkey. *Fed. Proc. 1:*51.

Merzenich, M. M., and Brugge, J. F. 1973. Representation of the cochlear partition on the superior temporal plane of the macaque monkey. *Brain Res. 50:*275–296.

Mesulam, M. M., and Pandya, D. N. 1973. The projections of the medial geniculate complex within the Sylvian fissure of the rhesus monkey. *Brain Res. 60:*315–333.

Moore, R. Y., and Goldberg, J. M. 1963. Ascending projections of the inferior colliculus in the cat. *J. Comp. Neurol. 121:*109–136.

Moore, R. Y., and Goldberg, J. M. 1966. Projections of the inferior colliculus in the monkey. *Exp. Neurol. 14:*429–438.

Moore, J. K., and Moore, R. Y. 1971. A comparative study of the superior olivary complex in the primate brain. *Folia Primatol. 16:*35–51.

Morest, D. K. 1964. The neuronal architecture of the medial geniculate body of the cat. *J. Anat. 98:*611–630.

Morest, D. K. 1965. The lateral tegmental system of the midbrain and the medial geniculate body: Study with Golgi and Nauta methods in cat. *J. Anat. 99:*611–634.

Moscowitz, N. 1969. Comparative aspects of some features of the central auditory system of primates. *Ann. N.Y. Acad. Sci. 167:*357–369.

Moscowitz, N., and Liu, J. 1972. Central projections of the spiral ganglion of the squirrel monkey. *J. Comp. Neurol. 144:*335–344.

Nauta, W. J. H., and Gygax, P. A. 1954. Silver impregnation of degenerating axons in the central nervous system: A modified technic. *Stain Technol. 29:*91–93.

Neff, W. D. 1961. Neural mechanisms of auditory discrimination. *In* W. A. Rosenblith (ed.). *Sensory Communication.* John Wiley, New York. Pp. 259–278.

Neff, W. D., Diamond, I. T., and Casseday, J. H. 1975. Behavioral studies of auditory discrimination: Central nervous system. *In* W. D. Keidel and W. D. Neff (eds.). *Handbook of Sensory Physiology, V: Auditory System.* Springer-Verlag, Berlin. Pp. 307–400.

Olszewski, J., and Baxter, D. 1954. *Cytoarchitecture of the Human Brain Stem.* J. P. Lippincott, Philadelphia. 199 pp.

Osen, K. K. 1969. Cytoarchitecture of the cochlear nuclei in the cat. *J. Comp. Neurol. 136:*453–484.

Papez, J. W. 1930. Superior olivary nucleus. Its fiber connections. *Arch. Neurol. Psychiatry 24:*1–20.

Penfield, W., and Perot, P. 1963. The brain's record of auditory and visual experience. *Brain 86:*595–697.

Poliak, S. 1932. The main afferent fiber systems of the cerebral cortex in primates. An investigation of the somato-sensory, auditory and visual paths of the cerebral cortex, with consideration of their normal and pathological function, based on experiments with monkeys. *In* H. M. Evans and I. M. Thompson (eds.). *University of California Publications in Anatomy.* University of California Press, Berkeley. Pp. 81–101.

Ramón y Cajal, S. 1909. *Histologie du système nerveux de l'homme et des vertébrés.* Vol. I. Reprinted 1955. Instituto Ramón y Cajal, Madrid. 986 pp.

Ramón y Cajal, S. 1911. *Histologie du système nerveux de l'homme et des vertébrés.* Vol. II. Reprinted 1955, Instituto Ramón y Cajal, Madrid. 993 pp.

Rasmussen, G. L. 1946. The olivary peduncle and other fiber projections of the superior olivary complex. *J. Comp. Neurol. 84:*141–219.

Rasmussen, G. L. 1960. Efferent fibers of the cochlear nerve and cochlear nucleus. *In* G. L. Rasmussen and W. F. Windle (eds.). *Neural Mechanisms of the Auditory and Vestibular Systems.* Charles C Thomas, Springfield. Pp. 105–115.

Rasmussen, G. L. 1964. Anatomic relationships of the ascending and descending auditory systems. *In* W. S. Fields and B. R. Alford (eds.). *Neurological Aspects of Auditory and Vestibular Disorders.* Charles C Thomas, Springfield. Pp. 5–19.

Rose, J. E. 1949. The cellular structure of the auditory region of the cat. *J. Comp. Neurol. 91:*409–440.

Rose, J. E., and Woolsey, C. N. 1949. The relations of thalamic connections, cellular structure and evocable electrical activity in the auditory region of the cat. *J. Comp. Neurol. 91:*441–466.

Rose, J. E., and Woolsey, C. N. 1958. Cortical connections and functional organization of the thalamic auditory system of the cat. *In* H. F. Harlow and C. N. Woolsey (eds.). *Biological and Biochemical Bases of Behavior.* University of Wisconsin, Madison. Pp. 127–150.

Rose, J. E., Galambos, R., and Hughes, J. 1959. Microelectrode studies of the cochlear nuclei of the cat. *Bull. Johns Hopkins Hosp. 104:*211–251.

Rose, J. E., Galambos, R., and Hughes, J. 1960. Organization of frequency sensitive neurons in the cochlear complex of the cat. *In* G. Rasmussen and W. Windle (eds.). *Mechanisms of the Auditory and Vestibular Systems.* Charles C Thomas, Springfield. Pp. 116–136.

Sanides, F. 1972. Representation in the cerebral cortex and its areal lamination patterns. *In* G. H. Bourne (ed.). *Structure and Function of Nervous Tissue,* Vol. 5. Academic Press, New York. Pp. 329–453.

Smith, C. A., and Rasmussen, G. L. 1965. Degeneration in the efferent nerve endings in the cochlea after axonal section. *J. Cell. Biol. 26:*63–77.

Sousa-Pinto, A. 1973. Cortical projections of the medial geniculate body in the cat. *Adv. Anat. Embryol. Cell Biol. 48:*1–42.

Spoendlin, H. H., and Gacek, R. R. 1963. Electronmicroscopic study of the efferent and afferent innervation of the organ of Corti in the cat. *Ann. Otol. Rhinol. Laryngol. 72:*660–686.

Stotler, W. A. 1953. An experimental study of the cells and connections of the superior olivary complex of the cat. *J. Comp. Neurol. 98:*401–431.

Stotler, W. A. 1957. A comparison of the cochlear nuclei of the primate and carnivore brainstem. *Anat. Rec. 127:*374.

Strominger, N. L. 1973. The origins, course and distribution of the dorsal and intermediate acoustic striae in the rhesus monkey. *J. Comp. Neurol. 147:*209–234.

Strominger, N. L., and Hurwitz, J. L. 1976. Anatomical aspects of the superior olivary complex. *J. Comp. Neurol. 170:*485–498.

Strominger, N. L., and Strominger, A. I. 1971. Ascending brain stem projections of the anteroventral cochlear nucleus in the rhesus monkey. *J. Comp. Neurol. 143:*217–242.

Strominger, N. L., Nelson, L. R., and Dougherty, W. J. 1977. Second order auditory pathways in the chimpanzee. *J. Comp. Neurol. 172:*349–366.

Strominger, N. L., Oesterreich, R. E., and Neff, W. D. 1978. Sequential auditory and visual discriminations after temporal lobe ablation in monkey. Unpublished manuscript.

Van Noort, J. 1969. *The Structure and Connections of the Inferior Colliculus. An Investigation of the Lower Auditory System.* Van Gorcum, Assen. 118 pp.

Walker, A. E. 1937. The projection of the medial geniculate body to the cerebral cortex in the macaque monkey. *J. Anat. 71:*319–331.

Walzl, E. M. 1947. Representation of the cochlea in the cerebral cortex. *Laryngoscope 57:*778–787.

Walzl, E. M., and Woolsey, C. N. 1943. Cortical auditory areas of the monkey as determined by electrical excitation of nerve fibers in the osseus spiral lamina and by click stimulation. *Fed. Proc. 2:*52.

Wegener, J. G. 1976. Auditory and visual discrimination following lesions of the anterior supratemporal plane in monkeys. *Neuropsychologia 14:*161–173.

Woolsey, C. N. 1960. Organization of cortical auditory system: A review and a synthesis. *In* G. L. Rasmussen and W. F. Windle (eds.). *Neural Mechanisms of the Auditory and Vestibular Systems*. Charles C Thomas, Springfield. Pp. 165–180.

Woolsey, C. N. 1972. Tonotopic organization of the auditory cortex. *In* M. B. Sachs (ed.). *Physiology of the Auditory System*. National Education Consultants, Baltimore. Pp. 271–282.

Woolsey, C. N., and Fairman, D. 1946. Contralateral, ipsilateral, and bilateral representation of cutaneous receptors in somatic areas I and II of the cerebral cortex of pig, sheep, and other mammals. *Surgery 19:*684–702.

Woolsey, C. N., and Walzl, E. M. 1944. Topical projection of the cochlea to the cerebral cortex of the monkey. *Am. J. Med. Sci. 207:*685–686.

4

Vocal Communication in Primates

LEONARD M. EISENMAN

I. Introduction

The living primates are social mammals that exhibit a variety of complex and subtle behavior patterns employing intricate communication systems. These patterns are expressions that have evolved during the long phylogenetic history of the various primate groups. The communication systems have utilized the auditory, visual, tactile, gustatory, and olfactory senses as essential modalities in the development, maintenance, and evolution of the social interactions in these primates. Attention in this discussion is directed to some recent findings, concepts, and speculations concerning the auditory aspects in the communication systems of several primates. These comprise (1) the auditory signal, including such aspects as vocalization repertoires, neural correlates, and ontogeny and (2) the perception of vocalization, including auditory sensitivity and the response properties of single neurons. The implications regarding the encoding of vocalizations by the nervous system are reviewed and discussed.

LEONARD M. EISENMAN • Department of Anatomy, Thomas Jefferson University, Philadelphia, Pennsylvania 19107.

It is critical to realize that communication behavior in primates is multimodal, i.e., it generally involves more than one sensory modality. In addition the communicative act(s) appears as part of a behavioral continuum and is dependent on physiological, environmental, and temporal factors (Schleidt, 1973). Removal of the auditory component of a multimodal communication signal for analysis is justified, but final evaluations and interpretations concerning the meaning of these auditory signals should be held in abeyance until the entire behavioral context is considered.

II. The Auditory Signal

A. Vocalization Repertoires

Vocal utterances constitute the largest class of auditory signals employed by primates in the communication process. The following account will focus on this category of auditory signal.

Primate vocalizations can vary one from the other in all auditory parameters, such as frequency, frequency modulation, amplitude, amplitude modulation, and duration. Attempts to categorize individual vocalizations of primate species based on these parametric differences have led to the formulation that individual primate species possess one of two types of vocalization repertoires (Marler, 1965). In the first, called the discrete vocalization system, individual vocalizations can be easily categorized or grouped according to one or more of the spectral parameters mentioned above. Few or no intermediates are apparent between these groupings. The size of the repertoire can be readily determined. As an example, Winter *et al.* (1966) describe 26 vocalizations in the squirrel monkey (*Saimiri sciureus*); these are classified into six groups. In the second, called the graded vocalization system, the vocalizations are not classifiable into precise subgroups because they seem to be distributed along a continuum. In an example typical for graded systems, Marler (1970) describes one basic pattern with variations as accounting for all of the vocalizations of the red colobus monkey (*Colobus badius*).

In terms of functional adaptation, the type of vocalization system (graded or discrete) a species utilizes appears to be important. Such primates as howler monkeys (*Cebus*), squirrel monkeys, and other species which inhabit forest areas (Marler, 1965, 1970; Worden and Galambos, 1972; Ploog, 1969) utilize discrete vocal systems. This is a habitat where visibility is poor, the noise level is high, and cohabitation with other species usually occurs. In contrast, a graded system of vocalization is used by the primarily land-dwelling species such as macaques and baboons. In this more open environment there is better visibility, less noise, and greater species isolation. Thus the vocal signal can usually be accompanied by a signal of a second sensory modality (e.g., visual), thereby presumably allowing greater subtleties of communication with little signal confusion.

Other significant factors compatible with the development of either graded or discrete systems are revealed in comparative studies of the red colobus (*C. badius*, Marler, 1970) and black and white colobus (*Colobus guereza*, Marler, 1972) monkeys. The red colobus is found to have a graded system whereas the black and white colobus exhibits a more discrete system even though they inhabit similar ecological areas. In these cases Marler suggests a number of species differences which might account for this distinction in their vocal repertoires. He notes that the troop size for the red colobus monkey (graded vocalizations) is three to five times greater than that for the black and white colobus monkey (discrete vocalizations). He then suggests that this difference is accompanied by a change in the emphasis from *inter*troop communication in the black and white colobus to *intra*troop communication in the red colobus monkey. Positive correlations are also found between the larynx size and communication distance. The black and white colobus monkey engages in more *inter*troop communication and presumably over greater distances; in addition, this species has a larger larynx than the red colobus monkey (Hill and Booth, 1957).

The use of either a discrete or graded vocalization system may be an adaptation by the species to its social structure and ecological niche. The main conclusions are that discrete systems provide better and more accurate distance communication between troops and are found also where species specificity is important or where visibility is poor. In contrast, graded vocalization systems may provide a richer and more subtle variety of signals especially when other sensory signals are given simultaneously.

Two other questions remain. First, can the varieties of graded signals be critically discriminated and discerned by the receiving animal? Initial evidence to be discussed later suggests that the acute ability to discriminate is present. Second, do animals respond to graded signals differentially if they can detect variations in graded signals? This question has not been satisfactorily handled as yet. In the study of this interpretative aspect of vocal signals, cognizance must be taken of the fact that all elements of the signal complex may be crucial, and the removal of one, in this case the vocal component, for analysis may result in mistaken interpretations as to the meaning of the entire signal.

B. Neural Correlates of Vocalizations

In attempts to identify the neural substrates involved with vocalization behavior, both ablation and stimulation studies have been performed. Several studies have been made of electrically stimulating areas of motor cortex representing face, tongue, and larynx in anesthetized macaque (*Macaca mulatta*) monkeys (Sugar *et al.*, 1948; Walker and Green, 1938; Robinson, 1967). Each of these experiments failed to elicit any vocalizations, natural or otherwise. Although vocalizations were not obtained in these stimulation studies, movements of the vocal cords were sometimes elicited. Jürgens (1974) repeated these experiments in squirrel monkeys by stimulating similar areas in both anesthetized and unanesthetized animals. In both of these experiments vocal cord movements were evoked, but vocalizations could not be elicited even in the unanesthetized monkey. Consistent with these findings was the report that bilateral ablation of these cortical areas in the macaque monkey did not result in loss of ability to vocalize (Myers, 1969).

In a series of studies, Jürgens and his collaborators (Jürgens, 1969; Jürgens and Ploog, 1970; Jürgens *et al.*, 1967) stimulated other regions of the squirrel monkey brain including those areas associated with the limbic system—the limbic lobe, thalamus, hypothalamus, and midbrain. Such stimulations produced vocalizations in unanesthetized squirrel monkeys. Similar results were obtained following stimulation of these structures in the unanesthetized (Robinson, 1967) and lightly anesthetized (Smith, 1941; Sloan and Kaada, 1953) rhesus monkey. Stimulation of these neural areas evoked responses in addition to vocalizations. These included such autonomic activities as penile erection, respiratory changes, or salivation. Because the accompanying evoked behavioral components were not always the same, attempted correlations between the vocalizations and the other behavioral responses is difficult.

In a recent study Sutton *et al.* (1974) made some relevant observations on macaque monkeys following the ablation of several cortical areas. They reported that these ablations differentially affected the performance of a trained prolonged vocalization. After bilateral removal of temporal association cortex or of the homologue of Broca's area or of transitional parietooccipital cortex no effect was evident on the postoperative performance of the vocalization. On the other hand, bilateral removal of the anterior cingulate and subcallosal areas resulted in a loss of the discriminative vocalization.

It appears clear, both from stimulation experiments and ablation studies, that the neural substrate for vocalization behavior is quite different in man than in the monkeys studied. In man, cortical areas in and around the triangular and opercular areas of the inferior frontal gyrus appear to be critically involved with vocalization behavior. In the monkey, the transitional cortex and subcortical areas related to the limbic system are the critical neural areas involved in this behavior.

Although the evidence is somewhat controversial, some work which has been done on the chimpanzee may be illuminating. Stimulation of cortical areas such as premotor cortex (Leyton and Sherrington, 1917; Dusser de Barenne *et al.,* 1941) and area 4 (Hines, 1940) in the chimpanzee did on occasion elicit vocalizations in this hominoid species. It appears clear that the important neural areas for vocalization behavior in different primates are not the same. There may have been an evolutionary progression from subcortical control of vocalization behavior in phylogenetically older primate species such as the squirrel monkey and rhesus monkey to increased cortical control in more recently evolved species such as chimpanzee and man. There is evidence which indicates that subcortical control over some aspects of vocalization behavior in man is still retained (Myers, 1969).

In many cases, the neural areas which are important in the production of vocalizations in nonhuman primates are also involved with emotional, motivational, and autonomic aspects of behavior. Marler (1965) points out that many vocalizations in nonhuman primates are related to the communication of "mood" or "change in mood"; this is a form of self-oriented communication. In man, communication systems seem to have evolved into more object-oriented vocal behavior. The neural substrates reflect these differences in communication systems.

The precise role of the cortical motor areas in the production of laryngeal movements in monkeys has yet to be determined. Jürgens (1974) suggests that these areas may have an important role in the "formation of new calls, either by learning from conspecifics or by matching to an innate auditory template." This does not seem to apply to the squirrel monkey for, as Winter *et al.* (1973) have argued, the vocal behavior in this monkey is innate, requiring no learning or auditory feedback. This will be discussed below.

C. Ontogeny of Vocalizations

Only a few experimental studies have been directed at analyzing the ontogeny of vocalizations in primates (Lenneberg, 1974). Most of the work has been done with the squirrel monkey and has indicated that the discrete cell system of this species is innate. Studies by Ploog *et al.* (1967), Talmage-Riggs *et al.* (1972), and Winter *et al.* (1973) demonstrate that neither auditory feedback nor matching of a model (a call uttered by another animal of the species) is necessary for the calls to develop. Some calls appear on the first day of life while other calls are not emitted until several days after birth. Ploog *et al.* (1967) suggest that the latter utterances may require certain correct conditions or may be dependent on maturational factors. Although the evidence seems convincing one small flaw remains. The earliest any animal was deafened to prevent auditory feedback was the fifth day of life. It appears that most, if not all, of the calls have appeared by this time. Therefore in order to rule out the contribution of auditory feedback as a factor in call development, experiments with deaf animals should be carried out in newborn squirrel monkeys (i.e., deafened as soon after birth as possible). This same procedure should be used to test the viability of Jürgens's (1974) suggestion that the neocortical areas which when stimulated produce laryngeal movements have a role in the learning or matching of calls. The evidence from the other studies cited above seems more in favor of the innateness of squirrel monkey vocalizations, and therefore some other unknown function may be served by these neocortical areas.

In a recent paper, Newman and Symmes (1974a) report the effects of social deprivation on the vocalization behavior of rhesus monkeys (*M. mulatta*). Rhesus monkeys were reared in isolation from birth to one month of age. There was no visual or auditory contact with other macaques, and the animals were minimally handled by human attendants. After the one month, the animals were placed in individual cages; this permitted visual and auditory contact with macaques of all ages. Newman and Symmes (1974a) report that these socially deprived monkeys exhibited structural abnormalities in their "clear" calls. However all other calls in these monkeys were similar to those in the control group.

This study, in contrast to those of the squirrel monkey, suggests that early manipulation of the social environment does affect the vocalization of the rhesus monkey, a species with a graded vocalization system (Rowell, 1962). It may be postulated that this graded system may have a different maturational course during ontogeny than have the discrete systems. The former is thought to possess more subtleties and variations which may depend more on experiential rather than genetic factors.

III. Perception of Vocalizations

A. Auditory Sensitivity

Up to this point, this review has dealt with the production of vocalizations. An equally important aspect of communication is the perception and recognition of these signals.

The auditory sensitivity of several primates has recently been studied by Stebbins (1973), Masterton et al. (1969), Heffner and Masterton (1970), Heffner et al. (1969), and Gillette et al. (1973). Comparative studies indicate that most nonhuman primates can hear a wider range of frequencies and are more sensitive to higher frequencies than is man. Based on the observations noted below, Masterton et al. (1969) suggest that during the evolution of primates (and more generally, mammals) there was a narrowing of the hearing range with a gradual reduction and loss in higher-frequency hearing.

Lemur catta has a high-frequency sensitivity up to 60 kHz (Gillette et al., 1973). This is essentially similar to that observed in the prosimian Galago senegalensis (Heffner et al., 1969) but higher than the 40-kHz sensitivity in the other prosimians Nycticebus coucang and Perodicticus potto (Heffner and Masterton, 1970). Other evidence indicates that anthropoidea such as cercopithecine monkeys (Stebbins, 1973) and chimpanzee (Stebbins, 1970) are sensitive to frequencies up to 40–45 kHz and 30 kHz, respectively. On the other hand, man is sensitive to frequencies up to about 20 kHz.

These differences in high-frequency sensitivity are probably not related to the perception of vocalizations because most primate vocalizations consist of frequencies below 20 kHz and most have their greatest energies below 4 or 5 kHz (Marler, 1965). Some components of prosimian vocalizations may have energies in the 25 to 30 kHz range, but here too the major energies are in the 10 to 15 kHz range (Gillette *et al.*, 1973). Masterton *et al.* (1969) argue that this change in auditory sensitivity is more probably related to sound localizing ability. Phylogenetically, as the mammalian head became larger, the mammal became less dependent on interaural intensity differences (i.e., the difference in the intensity of a sound at the two ears which results from the head acting as a sound shadow) as cues for sound localization. Instead, interaural time difference (Δt) became a more important cue for an animal with a large head.

Since high frequencies produce confusing Δt cues, the animal would probably be more dependent on the Δt cues resulting from the low-frequency components of sound stimuli. Therefore, high-frequency sensitivity could be sacrificed with no apparent loss in sound localizing ability (Masterton *et al.*, 1969).

Comparative observations on four different primates suggest that the perception of vocalizations may be related to the sensitivity to different frequencies. In contrast to man's relative sensitivity to different frequencies which begins to increase after 4 kHz, the threshold in nonhuman primates does not increase significantly (except for the chimpanzee) until about 25 kHz (Gillette *et al.*, 1973). Perhaps the low threshold to this higher frequency range (8–25 kHz) is related to the vocalization energies emitted by these species. Because vocalizations have important biological significance it would be extremely beneficial for an animal to have low absolute thresholds for the frequencies incorporated in its vocalization repertoire.

B. Responses of Single Auditory Neurons

In order to analyze another parameter associated with the perception of vocalizations, experiments have been performed to study the responses of single neurons in the auditory cortex to species-specific vocalizations. Again most of these studies have been performed on the squirrel monkey (*S. sciureus*), a primate with a discrete vocalization repertoire. The responses of cortical cells in the primary auditory area in unanesthetized squirrel monkeys to both simple acoustical signals (tone pips, clicks, and noise bursts) and also to species-specific vocalizations (Funkenstein and Winter, 1973) were recorded. Of the 283 cells which were monitored, 41% showed some response to vocalizations. Of these neurons, 48 were monitored extensively and form the substance of their study. In an attempt to classify the responses of these neurons it was found that cells differed greatly in terms of the calls to which they responded. The majority of the neurons (28, or 58%) appeared to respond only to one or two call types. These call types usually exhibited similar acoustic properties, i.e., mainly high- or low-frequency or noise components.

Because many of the neuronal units responded to both simple acoustic stimuli and to one or more calls, Winter and Funkenstein (1973) attempted to determine the predictability of a unit's response to calls based on its response to the simpler stimuli. Predictability was based on the unit's pure-tone response area and its response or lack of response to white noise. They reported that 30 cells (63%) exhibited predictable responses. The remaining neurons were "unpredictable" in that they responded to calls which contained frequencies outside their pure-tone response areas or they responded to neither tones nor noise but did show responses to calls. These latter neurons were termed "selective responders," in that they responded only to calls and indeed only to one or two types of calls.

At about this time Wollberg and Newman (1972; Newman and Wollberg, 1973a) studied the responses of cortical neurons in the same species to 12 species-specific vocalizations. They reported that 75 (90%) of the units studied with all 12 vocalizations responded to at least one of the calls. Unlike the results reported by Winter and Fuckenstein (1973), however, almost all (89%) of the cells responded to more than half of the vocalizations with which they were tested. The temporal patterns of the responses of a typical cell differed for different calls. In addition presentation of the same call produced many different temporal patterns of response in different cells. Therefore these authors suggested that a particular call did not seem to be represented by a unique temporal pattern of discharge. They noted that a unit's responses to different vocalizations were not predictable when predictability was based on their responses to simpler stimuli. This differed from the observations reported by Winter and Funkenstein (1973) noted above. One of the points of agreement in the studies was the finding that some cells would discriminate (in terms of responding or not responding) between calls which were acoustically similar but would not discriminate between calls which were apparently acoustically dissimilar. The crucial problem in these observations is to determine what features of the acoustic stimulus are critical in determining a neuron's response. The similarities between two stimuli which we hear or see (on a sound spectrograph) may be based on features of the stimulus which are unimportant in determing a neuron's response.

In a further study of this point Newman and Wollberg (1973b) studied the response of neurons to variations of one call type—the so-called "isolation peep." This call is apparently used when an individual loses contact with its troop, and the animal emits this vocalization in an attempt to regain contact. Seven variations of this call and two "atypical" variations of the call, in addition to representative examples of other call types, were used as stimuli. The authors found that most (21, or 57%) of the cells responded to all nine variations of the isolation peep and 19% responded to all seven typical variations but not to the atypical isolation peep calls. They also point out that a single neuron's temporal pattern of response to each variation was usually different. On the basis of these data the authors suggest that "many neurons in auditory cortex tend to categorize isolation peeps together" (Newman and Wollberg, 1973b).

The remaining neurons (24%) did *not* respond to all variants of the call but showed preferential responsiveness to some of the variants. The authors point out that they were unable to categorize, by the use of simple acoustic features, subgroups of the isolation peeps which had been responded to selectively. In a corresponding behavioral study, Symmes and Newman (1974) report that squirrel monkeys can behaviorally discriminate between these variations of the isolation peep call. Newman and Wollberg (1973b) suggest that the neurons which respond only to some of the variants and not others provide a mechanism by which behavioral discriminations can be made.

In an attempt to determine how other variables, besides the physical stimulus itself, affect the neuron's response, Newman and Symmes (1974b) studied the responses of cells in the auditory cortex of the squirrel monkey to stimulation of the midbrain reticular formation (RF) alone and simultaneously with presentation of a species-specific vocalization. The authors suggest that RF stimulation might serve as a substitute for spontaneously occurring shifts in the animal of such variables as attention and arousal.

Their findings indicate that some of the neurons (14 of 55) responded to RF stimulation alone. Thirty-nine neurons responded to species-specific vocalizations when these were presented alone. When RF stimulation was presented simultaneously with a species-specific call, 15 of these 39 neurons showed changes in response strength or response pattern. They also report that 4 of these neurons altered their selectivity to vocalizations when RF stimulation was presented concurrently. Of interest is the observation that of the 15 cells which altered their response to calls in the presence of RF stimulation, 9 of these neurons did not respond to RF stimulation alone. It appears as though these neurons in auditory cortex are in the "subliminal fringe" of the reticular neurons being stimulated. This concept was used by Lloyd (1943) to describe the monosynaptic effect of Ia afferents on motor neurons. The reticular formation apparently has a modulating influence on the activity of auditory cortical neurons. This is probably only one of many areas of the brain which has this type of modulating influence on the auditory cortex. The response of a neuron to a stimulus at any point in time would represent not only the effect of the stimulus but also the other modulating inputs which probably represent the general state (internal and external) of the animal.

Newman and Symmes (1974b) also found that there was no shift in selectivity to vocalizations with spontaneous changes in arousal as measured by cortical EEG. On the basis of these data the authors conclude that the coding properties of auditory cortical neurons do not change as a result of variations in spontaneous and/or RF-activated arousal.

However, these conclusions do not take into account the changes in the magnitude and/or the temporal pattern of a neuron's response to alterations in arousal. Newman and Symmes are probably correct in concluding that a neuron's "specificity" as measured in terms of responding or not responding would not be altered with changes in these variables. It is surprising to see those few neurons which did. However, it should be noted that in the responses of the neuron reported by them, the change in selectivity was the addition of other calls which could now evoke a response when presented simultaneously with RF stimulation. In other words the neuron's tuning to vocalizations becomes broader.

The general conclusion to be drawn from these studies is that auditory cortical neurons are for the most part not "specific" or narrowly tuned to vocalizations but rather broadly tuned to these sound stimuli. But it should be emphasized that although a neuron may respond to many calls it usually responds differentially to these calls in terms of temporal pattern and/or magnitude of the response. It is this differential sensitivity to vocalizations and to other variables present at the time of the communication which permits each vocalization and its attendant context to be uniquely and unambiguously encoded. This is most likely not accomplished by single "specific" neurons but more probably by an ensemble of differentially sensitive neurons (Erickson, 1968, 1974; Eisenman, 1974).

IV. Conclusions and Summary

Some of the more recent studies relevant to the production and reception of vocalizations used by nonhuman primates as part of their communication systems have been reviewed. Intriguing questions have been raised, which, it is hoped, will guide future research.

In summary, there are two basic types of vocalization repertoires, discrete systems and graded systems. The discrete systems are usually associated with phylogenetically older primates while the graded systems are found in the more recently evolved species. There does seem to be some overlap between the two groups. It would be interesting to determine whether the graded system is the more intricate communication system and whether it might be an expression of an intermediate stage between the discrete systems and human language.

The neural correlates of primate vocalizations appear to be different in man from those of other primates. Vocalizations in the latter appear to be associated with limbic and midbrain structures with a minimum of cortical influences. In contrast, vocalizations in man seem to be predominantly influenced by cortical activity. These differences appear to correlate with the "self-oriented" and "object-oriented" communications of nonhuman primates and man, respectively (Marler, 1965).

The ontogeny of vocalization has been primarily studied in the squirrel monkey. In this species the repertoire appears to be genetically determined with few, if any, environmental influences. The notion that species with graded systems may follow a different ontogenetic course has been presented.

The auditory sensitivity of primates has been reviewed with perhaps the main observation being that "more recently evolved species" are not sensitive to frequencies above 20 to 40 kHz. This is apparently not related to the perception of vocalizations, as the frequencies used by these species in vocalizing are in lower ranges. The suggestion was made that a correlation may exist between the relative sensitivity to frequency and the frequencies used by a species in its vocalizations. However, this remains to be documented.

The study of the responses of single auditory cortical neurons has shown that the majority of these neurons are broadly tuned to vocalizations. Individual vocalizations are probably encoded at this stage of the auditory system by populations of differentially sensitive neurons. All of these studies were done with the squirrel monkey, which was a discrete vocalization system; thus it remains to be determined what the neuronal responses are in a primate with a graded system of vocalizations.

In reviewing the auditory communication of primates it is difficult to avoid the impression that the continuing evolution of this order of mammals has, in part, involved the transition from a fixed, species-specific, genetically determined system of vocalizations to a more flexible, intricate, environmentally influenced system. However, much information remains to be obtained before the details of the evolutionary transitions become clear.

Acknowledgment.   It is a pleasure to thank Dr. Charles R. Noback for his helpful suggestions and critical reading of the manuscript.

V. References

Dusser de Barenne, J. G., Carol, H. W., and McCulloch, W. S. 1941. The "motor" cortex of the chimpanzee. *J. Neurophysiol. 4:*287–303.

Eisenman, L. M. 1974. Neural encoding of sound location: An electro-physiological study in auditory cortex of the cat using free field stimuli. *Brain Res. 75:*203–214.

Erickson, R. P. 1968. Stimulus coding in topographic and nontopographic modalities: On the significance of the activity of individual sensory neurons. *Psychol. Rev. 75:*447–465.

Erickson, R. P. 1974. Parallel "population" neural coding in feature extraction. *In* F. O. Schmitt and F. G. Worden (eds.). *Neurosciences: A Third Study Program.* MIT Press, Cambridge. Pp. 155–170.

Funkenstein, H. H., and Winter, P. 1973. Responses to acoustic stimuli of units in auditory cortex of awake squirrel monkeys. *Exp. Brain Res. 18:*464–488.

Gillette, R. G., Brown, R., Herman, P., Vernon, S., and Vernon, J. 1973. The auditory sensitivity of the lemur. *Am. J. Phys. Anthropol. 38:*365–370.

Heffner, H., and Masterton, B. 1970. Hearing in primitive primates: Slow loris (*Nycticebus coucang*) and potto (*Perodicticus potto*). *J. Comp. Physiol. Psychol. 71:*175–182.

Heffner, H., Ravizza, R., and Masterton, B. 1969. Hearing in primitive mammals. IV: Bushbaby (*Galago senegalensis*). *J. Aud. Res. 9:*19–23.

Hill, W. C. O., and Booth, A. H. 1957. Voice and larynx in African and Asiatic colobidae. *J. Bombay Nat. Hist. Soc. 54:*309–321.

Hines, M. 1940. Movements elicited from precentral gyrus of adult chimpanzees by stimulation with sine wave currents. *J. Neurophysiol. 3:*442–466.

Jürgens, U. 1969. Correlation between brain structure and vocalization type elicited in the squirrel monkey. *In* H. O. Hofer (ed.). *Proc 2nd. Int. Congr. Primatol. Atlanta 1968,* Vol. 3. Karger, Basel. Pp. 28–33.

Jürgens, U. 1974. On the excitability of vocalization from the cortical larynx area. *Brain Res. 81:*564–566.

Jürgens, U., and Ploog, D. 1970. Cerebral representation of vocalization in the squirrel monkey. *Exp. Brain Res. 10:*532–554.

Jürgens, U., Maurus, M., Ploog, D., and Winter, P. 1967. Vocalizations in the squirrel monkey (*Saimiri sciureus*) elicited by brain stimulation. *Exp. Brain Res. 4:*114–117.

Lenneberg, E. H. 1974. Language and brain: Developmental aspects. *Neurosci. Res. Program, Bull. 12:*513–656.

Leyton, A. S. F., and Sherrington, C. S. 1917. Observations on the excitable cortex of the chimpanzee, orangutan and gorilla. *J. Exp. Physiol. 11:*135–222.

Lloyd, D. P. C. 1943. Reflex action in relation to pattern and peripheral source of afferent stimulation. *J. Neurophysiol. 6:*111–120.

Marler, P. 1965. Communication in monkeys and apes. *In* DeVore (ed.). *Primate Behavior: Field Studies of Monkeys and Apes.* Rinehart and Winston, New York. Pp. 544–584.

Marler, P. 1970. Vocalizations of East African monkeys. I. Red colobus. *Folia Primatol. 13:*81–91.

Marler, P. 1972. Vocalizations of East African monkeys. II: Black and white colobus. *Behaviour 42:*175–197.

Masterton, B., Heffner, H., and Ravizza, R. 1969. The evolution of human hearing. *J. Acoust. Soc. Am. 45:*966–985.

Myers, R. E. 1969. Neurology of social communication in primates. *In* H. O. Hofer (ed.). *Proc. 2nd Int. Congr. Primatol. Atlanta, 1968,* Vol 3. Karger, Basel. Pp. 1–9.

Newman, J. D., and Symmes, D. 1974a. Vocal pathology in socially deprived monkeys. *Dev. Psychobiol. 7:*351–358.

Newman, J. D., and Symmes, D. 1974b. Arousal effects of unit responsiveness to vocalizations in squirrel monkey auditory cortex. *Brain Res. 78:*125–138.

Newman, J. D., and Wollberg, Z. 1973a. Multiple coding of species specific vocalizations in auditory cortex of squirrel monkeys. *Brain Res. 54:*287–304.

Newman, J. D., and Wollberg, Z. 1973b. Responses of single neurons in auditory cortex of squirrel monkeys to varients of a single call type. *Exp. Neurol. 40:*821–824.

Ploog, D. 1969. Early communication processes in squirrel monkeys. *In* R. J. Robinson (ed.). *Brain and Early Behavior: Development in the Fetus and Infant.* Academic Press, New York. Pp. 269–298.

Ploog, D., Hopf, S., and Winter, P. 1967. Ontogenese des Verhaltens von Totenkopf-Affen (*Saimiri sciureus*). *Psychol. Forsch. 31:*1–41.

Robinson, B. W. 1967. Vocalization evoked from forebrain in *Macaca mulatta*. *Physiol. Behav. 2:*345–354.

Rowell, J. E. 1962. Agonistic noises of the rhesus monkey (*Macaca mulatta*). *Symp. Zool. Soc. London 8:*91–96.

Schleidt, W. M. 1973. Tonic communication: Continual effects of discrete signs in animal communication systems. *J. Theor. Biol. 42:*359–386.

Sloan, N., and Kaada, B. 1953. Efforts of anterior limbic stimulation on somato-motor and electro-cortical activity. *J. Neurophysiol. 16:*203–220.

Smith, W. K. 1941. Vocalization and other responses elicited by excitation of the regio cingularis in the monkey. *Am. J. Physiol. 133:*451–452.

Sugar, O., Chusid, J. G., and French, J. D. 1948. A second motor cortex in the monkey (*Macaca mulatta*). *J. Neuropathol. Exp. Neurol. 7:*182–189.

Stebbins, W. C. 1970. Hearing. *In* A. M. Schrier and F. Stollnitz (eds.). *Behavior of Non-human Primates,* Vol. 3. Academic Press, New York. Pp. 159–192.

Stebbins, W. C. 1973. Hearing of Old World monkeys (*Cercopithecinae*). *Am. J. Phys. Anthropol. 38:* 357–364.

Sutton, D., Larson, C., and Lindeman, R. C. 1974. Neocortical and limbic lesion effects on primate phonation. *Brain Res. 71:*61–75.

Symmes, D., and Newman, J. D. 1974. Discrimination of isolation prep varients by squirrel monkeys. *Exp. Brain Res. 19:*365–376.

Talmage-Riggs, G., Winter, P., Ploog, D., and Mayer, W. 1972. Effect of deafening on vocal behavior of the squirrel monkey (*Saimiri sciureus*). *Folio Primatol. 17:*404–420.

Walker, A. E., and Green, H. D. 1938. Electrical excitability of the motor face area: A comparative study in primates. *J. Neurophysiol. 1:*152–165.

Winter, P., and Funkenstein, H. H. 1973. The effect of species-specific vocalization on the discharge of auditory cortical cells in the awake squirrel monkey (*Saimiri sciureus*). *Exp. Brain Res. 18:*489–504.

Winter, P., Ploog, D., and Latta, J. 1966. Vocal repertoire of the squirrel monkey (*Saimiri sciureus*), its analysis and significance. *Exp. Brain Res. 1:*359–384.

Winter, P., Handley, P., Ploog, D., and Schott, D. 1973. Ontogeny of squirrel monkey calls under normal conditions and under acoustic isolation. *Behaviour 47:*230–239.

Wollberg, Z., and Newman, J. D. 1972. Auditory cortex of squirrel monkey: Response patterns of single cells to species-specific vocalizations. *Science 175:*212–214.

Worden, F. G., and Galambos, R. 1972. Auditory processing of biologically significant sounds. *Neurosci. Res. Program, Bull. 10:*1–119.

5

Structural and Functional Aspects of the Superior Colliculus in Primates

Roberta Pierson Pentney and John R. Cotter

I. Introduction

The superior colliculus is a phylogenetically old cortex, but determination and measurement of its function in primates has proved to be a particularly difficult and challenging task. It has been known for over a century that stimulation of the colliculus produces eye movements (Adamuk, 1870), but no experimental design has yielded an adequate answer to the question of the exact functional role of the colliculus.

An extensive review of current information concerning the mammalian superior colliculus with particular emphasis upon studies conducted in the domestic cat was published recently (Sprague *et al.*, 1973). A similar review emphasizing studies in primates has not been available. The purpose of this paper is to attempt to bring together in

Roberta Pierson Pentney and John R. Cotter • Department of Anatomical Sciences, State University of New York, Buffalo, New York 14214.

one short chapter the major pieces of information collected from studies of the superior colliculus of primates. We have not attempted to provide a complete review of the literature, and certain areas of investigation, described in detail elsewhere in this volume, are considered only briefly. The experimental results we shall consider have been arbitrarily grouped for ease of consideration under three headings: anatomical studies of cytoarchitecture and fiber connections, physiological studies of cellular activity, and behavioral studies.

II. Anatomical Studies

A. Cytoarchitecture

Ramón y Cajal's (1955) lucid descriptions and illustrations of the cytoarchitecture and fiber composition of the superior colliculus form the basis of our understanding of the mammalian tectum. Cajal's studies utilized cat, rabbit, and mouse tissues prepared according to the Golgi and Weigert methods. As yet there are no published Golgi studies of the primate superior colliculus, most likely due to the fact that adult tissues are often refractory to the Golgi stains. A recent modification of the Golgi procedure developed by Scheibel *et al.* (1973) for use with adult tissues should lead to such studies in the near future and provide us with a better understanding of the cytoarchitecture and organization of the primate tectum.

Ramón y Cajal (1955) divided the superior colliculus into five laminar zones: (1) a thin outer zone of fine tangential fibers lying above horizontal and piriform cells of average and small size; (2) a zone of vertically arranged diverse cell types each with dendrites directed radially toward the outer zone; (3) a zone of anteroposteriorly directed optic fiber bundles and large fusiform or stellate cells; (4) a wide ganglion layer containing average to large-sized cells scattered among transverse fiber bundles; and (5) a zone of central gray.

According to Ramón y Cajal's illustrations (1955) the dendrites of these various cell types are for the most part confined to their zone of origin. The majority of the axons, on the other hand, descend to join the fiber systems in the fourth zone, usually after giving rise to one or more recurrent collaterals. Many of the axons arise from a dendritic trunk rather than from the soma and arch upward before descending, forming what Cajal called a "shepherd's crook."

Various systems of nomenclature for the laminar pattern of the vertebrate tectum have been developed since Cajal's studies. These have been described in detail by Huber and Crosby (1933, 1943). The number of laminae designated morphologically has varied from two or three in urodeles to fifteen in birds, but when designated on the basis of both morphology and function a fundamental pattern of six strata or laminae emerges (Huber and Crosby, 1933) (Fig. 1). These are usually either numbered 1 through 6 as one proceeds from the collicular surface to deeper levels, or the laminae are named individually, according to appearance, position, or characteristic fiber connections. The stratum zonale (SZ), stratum cinereum or stratum griseum superficiale (SGS),

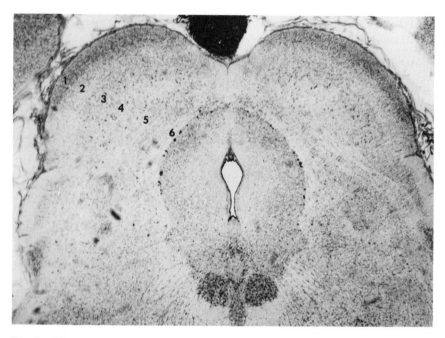

Fig. 1. Photomicrograph of the primate superior colliculus. In this transverse section through the midbrain of *Macaca mulatta*, the superior colliculus is found between the cerebral aqueduct and the dorsal surface of the brainstem. The six laminae of the superior colliculus are identified: (1) the stratum griseum superficiale; (2) the stratum opticum; (3) the stratum griseum intermediale; (4) the stratum album intermediale; (5) the stratum griseum profundum; (6) the stratum album profundum. The central gray encircles the aqueduct. Nissl stain. (Courtesy Dr. Norman Strominger.)

and stratum opticum (SO)—the first three strata—correspond to the
first three zones of Ramón y Cajal (1955). The ganglion zone of Ramón
y Cajal (1955) is further divided into the stratum griseum intermediale
(SGI), stratum album intermediale (SAI), stratum griseum profundum
(SGP), and stratum album profundum (SAP) (Huber and Crosby,
1943; Sprague, 1975; Williams and Warwick, 1975). Cajal's fifth zone,
the central gray, is omitted in this scheme of collicular organization
though the dendritic termination of some cells in the central gray jus-
tifies its inclusion in the tectum (Mehler, 1969; Sprague, 1975).

The descriptions of the primate superior colliculus have been based
chiefly on Weigert and Nissl preparations (Huber and Crosby, 1933;
Olszewski and Baxter, 1954; Oh, 1973). In a recent detailed study of
Nissl preparations of the superior colliculus in a number of primate
species (*Papio papio, Papio cynocephalus, Papio hamadryas, Macaca
mulatta, Macaca irus, Macaca sinca,* and *Cercopithecus aethiops*) Oh
(1973) described three major horizontal zones which he called the
external, intermediate, and internal zones. The external zone includes
the first three superficial strata designated by other investigators.
Within the external zone Oh (1973) found variations in cytoarchitecture
which could not be accounted for by species differences, e.g., *M. mulatta*
and *P. hamadryas* both have an almost cell-free surface zone while *P.
papio* and *P. cynocephalus* do not. With his limited material Oh (1973)
could only attribute such differences to individual variation. His intermediate zone includes the SGI and SAI, and his internal zone includes
the SGP and SAP (Oh, 1973).

The most detailed information regarding the cytoarchitecture of the
primate superior colliculus has resulted from the ultrastructural studies
of Lund (1972) in *M. mulatta* and Tigges, M., *et al.* (1973) in *Galago
crassicaudatus.* According to Lund (1972) the SZ can be identified by
light microscopy as a distinct layer, 10–15 μm in thickness. In this layer
myelinated axons are oriented tangentially to the collicular surface, but
the neuropil between these axons in electron micrographs appears
identical to that seen in the SGS. This suggests that there is no clear-cut
justification for differentiating these two regions as separate layers in
the monkey. He also found that a distinct layer of horizontal cells could
not be identified in the upper part of the SGS in monkey tissue as it
could in rat, rabbit, and cat tissues (Ramón y Cajal, 1955; Lund, 1969;
Sterling, 1971), but the basic synaptic patterns in the upper layers were
similar to those in rat and cat (Lund, 1969, 1970; Lund and Lund,

1971a,b; Sterling, 1971). Sterling (1971) suggested in an earlier study of the cat superior colliculus that Cajal's designation of a zone of horizontal cells and a zone of vertical cells in the SGS was misleading because the cells within these zones are not directed exclusively horizontally or vertically. But he could distinguish laminar subdivisions in the SGS based upon the extent of the dendritic arborizations at different levels in the SGS (Sterling, 1971).

With regard to synaptic patterns in the superficial layers of the monkey superior colliculus, Lund (1972) found that 95% of the synapses in his material were axodendritic. The remaining 5% consisted of serial synaptic patterns, involving axodendritic, dendrodendritic, and, rarely, axosomatic synapses between adjacent terminals. Two major types of terminals could be identified, one with round or spheroidal vesicles (S terminals) and one with flattened or pleomorphic vesicles (F terminals). S terminals could be subdivided further according to the electron density of their mitochondria, and F terminals according to the size and arrangement of their vesicles. Small S terminals with pale mitochondria located in the upper half of the SGS were identified experimentally as terminals of optic tract fibers whereas larger S terminals containing dark mitochondria corresponded to corticotectal terminations. Both types of S terminals appeared to be axonal and were always presynaptic (Lund, 1972).

A similar study of the normal patterns of synaptic organization in the superficial collicular layers in *Galago* was conducted by Tigges, M., *et al.* (1973). Three types of terminals designated as R1, R2, and F types were distinguished (Fig. 2). R1 terminals contained round vesicles, clustered only in part of the terminal, and relatively dark mitochondria in an electron lucent cytoplasm. R2 terminals contained round homogeneously distributed vesicles and pale mitochondria. F terminals with flat vesicles were quite numerous. R terminals were always presynaptic and presumed to originate from axons. F terminals were always postsynaptic to R terminals and could be postsynaptic to dendrites, other F profiles, and, rarely, to somata. The R1 and F terminals were found in all three of the superficial collicular layers, SZ, SGS, and SO. The R2 terminals were much more restricted in distribution and were located mainly in the upper and middle part of SGS. Following unilateral enucleation these latter terminals were identified as retinocollicular terminals. These authors did not attempt to identify the cortical terminals, but the general agreement of their results with those

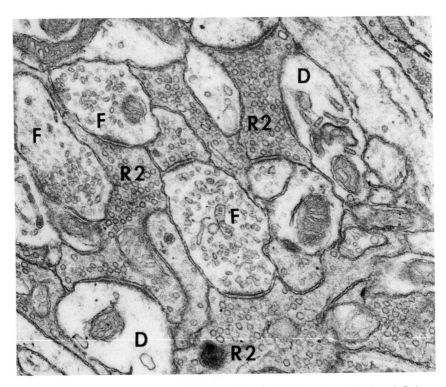

Fig. 2.   Different types of synapses in normal neuropil of superior colliculus of *Galago*. A cluster of R2 terminals making asymmetrical contacts with small dendritic profiles (D) and F profiles. ×48,000. (From Tigges, M., Tigges, J., Luttrell, G. L., and Frazier, C. M. 1973. *Z. Zellforsch. Mikrosk. Anat. 140*:291–307.)

of Lund (1972) would suggest that their R1 terminals may originate from corticocollicular fibers.

Future Golgi preparations will be essential in working out the source and relationships of the F terminals.

B. Fiber Connections

1. Retinotectal Projections.   In *Tupaia*, fibers of retinal origin project to the superior colliculus bilaterally and terminate in superficial and intermediate layers (Tigges, 1966; Campbell *et al.*, 1967; Laemle, 1968; Campbell, 1969; Giolli and Tigges, 1970). A small number of retinotectal fibers also terminate contralaterally in the SGP (Laemle,

1968). Ipsilaterally retinotectal terminations are located primarily in the SGI (Campbell *et al.*, 1967). The contralateral projection is larger and contains fibers from both nasal and temporal portions of the retina (Kaas *et al.*, 1974).

Retinotectal projections have been studied in a number of primate genera. Among these are *Galago* (Campos-Ortega and Clüver, 1968; Tigges and Tigges, 1970; Tigges, J., *et al.*, 1973), *Perodicticus* (Giolli and Tigges, 1970), *Nycticebus* (Campbell, 1969), *Saimiri* (Campos-Ortega and Glees, 1967a,b; Campbell, 1969; Tigges and Tigges, 1969; Tigges and O'steen, 1974), and *Macaca* (Hendrickson *et al.*, 1970; Wilson and Toyne, 1970; Pierson and Carpenter, 1974). As in *Tupaia* more fibers end on the contralateral side, but all fibers appear to terminate in the superficial layers.

Although the general pattern of retinotectal projections is similar in *Galago, Perodicticus, Saimiri,* and *Macaca*, the specific topographical pattern of terminations varies from species to species. For example, in *Galago*, retinal fibers terminate in three compartments or subdivisions of the SGS (Tigges and Tigges, 1970). The first of these zones of termination, substratum A, is located immediately beneath the SZ. Substratum C is located in the deepest sector of the superficial gray. Both substratum A and substratum C are regions of termination for fibers originating in the contralateral retina. Ipsilateral projections terminate in an area of the superficial gray between substrata A and C (substratum B) and also in substratum C. On the other hand, Giolli and Tigges (1970) identified only two levels of retinal termination within the SGS in *Perodicticus*. Substratum A, located in the upper half of the SGS, receives a contralateral projection, and substratum B, located in its lower half, receives ipsilateral fibers.

The termination of retinotectal fibers in the SGS is organized differently in *Saimiri* and *Macaca* (Hendrickson *et al.*, 1970; Wilson and Toyne, 1970; Tigges and O'steen, 1974). In *Saimiri*, terminals occur principally in the uppermost portion of this layer (Tigges and O'steen, 1974). In the macaque, the contralateral and ipsilateral retinal terminations are not uniformly distributed along the rostrocaudal extent of the colliculus (Hubel *et al.*, 1975). At the rostrolateral pole, the termination of projections from both eyes alternate with one another across the width of the colliculus. Further caudal contralateral and ipsilateral projections are segregated into dorsal and ventral compartments of the SGS respectively. In the caudomedial colliculus the projection is limited to the contralateral retina. In these two primates projection from the foveal part of the retina was believed to be substantially less than that of the peripheral retina (Hendrickson *et al.*, 1970; Wilson and Toyne, 1970; Pierson and Carpenter, 1974; Tigges and O'steen, 1974). Hubel *et al.* (1975) however have demonstrated the foveal projection in *Macaca*.

    2. Corticotectal Projections.   In the rhesus monkey the cerebral cortex gives rise to numerous efferents many of which terminate in the brain stem. Those which reach the colliculus, or corticotectal fibers as they are called, originate in frontal (Kuypers and Lawrence, 1967; Goldman and Nauta, 1976; Künzle *et al.*, 1976), parietal (Peele, 1942; Kuypers and Lawrence, 1967), temporal (Whitlock and Nauta, 1956; Kuypers and Lawrence, 1967), and occipital (Kuypers and Lawrence, 1967; Campos-Ortega *et al.*, 1970; Wilson and Toyne, 1970) cortices. Terminations in the colliculus are ipsilateral to their site of origin. Similar tectal projections may occur in primates other than the rhesus monkey but, as yet, only a projection from the occipital lobe has been identified in *Tupaia* (Abplanalp, 1970; Harting and Noback, 1971), *Galago* (Campos-Ortega, 1968; Tigges, J., *et al.*, 1973), and *Saimiri* (Spatz *et al.*,1970). This projection is topographically organized in the tree shrew (Abplanalp, 1970; Harting and Noback, 1971), squirrel monkey (Kadoya *et al.*, 1971a), and rhesus monkey (Wilson and Toyne, 1970). This projection may provide for overlap between occipitotectal and retinotectal systems at the level of the colliculus.

    Anatomic studies indicate that corticotectal projections terminate in specific laminae of the rhesus colliculus. Those arising from the visual cortex terminate primarily in the superficial layers (Kuypers and Lawrence, 1967; Campos-Ortega *et al.*, 1970; Wilson and Toyne, 1970). Far fewer fibers terminate in the SGI. The projection from this area of cortex is also limited in its termination to the superficial collicular layers in *Tupaia* (Abplanalp, 1971; Harting and Noback, 1971), *Galago* (Campos-Ortega, 1968), and *Saimiri* (Spatz *et al.*, 1970). While corticotectal projections from other cortical areas have not been studied in these primate forms, studies in the rhesus monkey (Peele, 1942; Whitlock and Nauta, 1956; Kuypers and Lawrence, 1967) suggest that frontal, temporal, and parietal projections terminate in the intermediate and deep strata of the primate colliculus. A projection from the prefrontal cortex to the SGI and SGP (Goldman and Nauta, 1976) and a projection from the frontal eye field to the SZ, SGS, SO, and SGI (Künzle *et al.*, 1976) were recently demonstrated. Corticomesencephalic afferents from precentral, postcentral, or parietal areas of the hemisphere (Kuypers and Lawrence, 1967) also project to the colliculus but terminate near its laterobasal border. An especially heavy projection to this region appears to arise from the lower parts of the postcentral and precentral gyrus. It may be that this region of the colliculus corresponds to Olszewski and Baxter's (1954) nucleus intercollicularis (Mehler, 1969).

The projection to the superior colliculus from cortical areas which are usually considered to have sensory and motor functions suggests that these aspects of cortical function may influence collicular neurons. The nature of the possible influence exerted by the occipital cortex was tested by recording from collicular neurons after removal or cooling of the visual cortex (Schiller *et al.*, 1974). In the superficial layers, the receptive field and response properties of collicular neurons were slightly altered by this procedure. Units in the superficial layers still responded, of course, because of the termination of the optic tract fibers in these laminae. Subtle changes in the properties of these neurons, as for example changes in attentional properties described by Goldberg and Wurtz (1972b), were not examined. More obvious changes were observed in the deeper layers. Here units which normally respond to visual stimuli failed to do so, but eye movement neurons were still encountered. Since the striate cortex processes visual information before the information is relayed to other areas, an important link by which visual information reaches the deep collicular layers appears to be disrupted by this procedure.

Recently, units recorded from area 7 of the cerebal cortex and units found at the border between superficial and intermediate collicular layers were shown to possess similar response characteristics, i.e., they discharge before saccadic eye movements and do not discharge during spontaneous saccades (Lynch *et al.*, 1975; Mohler and Wurtz, 1975). Lynch *et al.* (1975) propose that such cortical neurons initiate visually triggered saccades, and Mohler and Wurtz (1975) suggest that such collicular neurons form part of the motor outflow from the colliculus. Whether both neuronal types contribute to a single functional system has yet to be determined.

3. Other Tectal Afferents. It is clear from behavioral, electrophysiological, and anatomical studies in primates and other species that sensory afferents other than those of the visual system project to the tectum. In the monkey certain nonvisual afferents have been demonstrated. They include projections from sensory and motor cortex (Kuypers and Lawrence, 1967), the inferior colliculus (Moore and

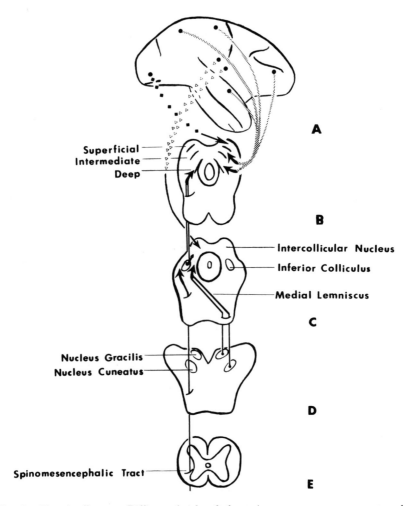

Fig. 3. Tectal afferents. Different levels of the primate nervous system are schematically illustrated. The cortical surface (A) is viewed from the lateral surface of the right cerebral hemisphere. The midbrain (B,C), medulla (D), and the spinal cord (E) are depicted in cross sections through each level. Corticotectal fibers originating in frontal, parietal, and temporal cortices (indicated by fine stipple) terminate in intermediate and deep laminae of the superior colliculus. Corticotectal fibers originating in visual cortex (indicated by solid blocks) terminate in the superficial laminae of the superior colliculus. Corticotectal fibers originating near the central fissure (indicated by open triangles) terminate in the intercollicular nucleus. Collaterals (indicated in solid lines) of the spinomesencephalic tract, medial lemniscus, and brachium of the inferior colliculus (not labeled) project to the intercollicular nucleus. Rostral continuations of the spinomesencephalic tract and brachium of the inferior colliculus also project to the deep laminae of the superior colliculus.

Goldberg, 1966), and the spinal cord (Mehler *et al.,* 1960; Mehler, 1969). Figure 3 illustrates the anatomical relationships of these afferents in the monkey. Also included in Fig. 3 are projections from the spinal cord and dorsal column nuclei which have been described in the tree shrew (Schroeder and Jane, 1971). In both species such nonvisual fiber systems project to collicular levels where they terminate especially in the region of the colliculus referred to as the intercollicular nucleus by Olszewski and Baxter (1954).

4. Tectal Efferents. Although ascending and descending tectal efferents terminate in a variety of brainstem nuclei (Myers, 1963; Harting *et al.,* 1973; Benevento and Fallon, 1975), they can be systematically organized according to their origin in either the superficial or deep laminae of the colliculus and the nuclei to which they project. Such a scheme has been identified in *Tupaia* (Casagrande *et al.,* 1972; Harting *et al.,* 1973) and *Macaca* (Benevento and Fallon, 1975) and may be present in *Galago* (Harting *et al.,* 1972). Other primate studies (Myers, 1963; Abplanalp, 1970, 1971; Mathers, 1971) have not investigated collicular efferents from this viewpoint.

The origin of tectal efferents from either superficial or deep layers of the colliculus and their projection to different brainstem nuclei make it possible to view the superior colliculus from the standpoint of two separate and perhaps independent anatomical and functional subdivisions (Casagrande *et al.,* 1972; Harting *et al.,* 1973). The superficial layers form in part a retino-tecto-pulvinar pathway which is considered to play an important role in pattern discrimination (Casagrande *et al.,* 1972). The role of the superficial layers in pattern discrimination other than that of a relay nucleus is however unclear. The deep layers, on the other hand, project to totally different nuclei among which are certain motor nuclei of the brain stem. Subsequent interconnections of these nuclei with the cerebellum, reticular formation, and motor neurons of the spinal cord may be the route by which the colliculus influences head and eye movements. For further details the reader is referred to Chapter 6 of this volume.

III. Physiological Studies

A. Visual Field Representation

A representation of the visual field upon the superior colliculus has been demonstrated electrophysiologically in the tree shrew (Lane *et al.,*

1971), the bush baby and owl monkey (Lane *et al.*, 1973), the squirrel monkey (Kadoya *et al.*, 1971b), and the rhesus monkey (Schiller and Koerner, 1971; Cynader and Berman, 1972; Goldberg and Wurtz, 1972a). The pattern of representation is built from the visual receptive fields of individual collicular neurons which are organized topographically across the colliculus. Receptive fields that include the center of gaze are represented in the rostral portion of the colliculus. Receptive fields recorded from this region of the colliculus are generally smaller than those recorded from the same lamina at more caudal levels. Occasionally foveal fields may also extend into or overlap the visual field ipsilateral to the recording site (Goldberg and Wurtz, 1972a; Lane *et al.*, 1973). Ipsilateral overlap that does occur (Humphrey, 1968; Cynader and Berman, 1972; Lane *et al.*, 1973) is more extensive in the deeper laminae.

The size of the receptive field increases with the depth at which recordings are made (Humphrey, 1968; Cynader and Berman, 1972; Goldberg and Wurtz, 1972a; Lane *et al.*, 1973). In the superficial layers field sizes may be less than 1° in size (Goldberg and Wurtz, 1972a; Cynader and Berman, 1972), but they may also be larger than 5° (Schiller and Koerner, 1971; Goldberg and Wurtz, 1972a). Receptive fields in the intermediate layers vary in size from 1–70°, and those of binocular neurons in the deeper layers are in some cases larger (Cynader and Berman, 1972). At rostral levels of the colliculus the trend toward receptive fields which are smaller than those at caudal levels continues in spite of increasing field sizes with the depth of recording. At both levels, when electrode advancements are perpendicular to the collicular surface, small receptive fields of the superficial layers occupy segments of visual space included in larger fields of the deeper layers (Goldberg and Wurtz, 1972a).

B. Unit Types in the Monkey Colliculus

1. Superficial Layers. Collicular neurons may respond to the presentation (onset), removal (offset), or to both onset and offset of a stationary spot of light. The receptive fields of such neurons are then said to be of the on, off, or on–off center type. Antagonistic or inhibitory surrounds may also be present.

Units responsive to stationary stimuli are contrasted with neurons whose discharge patterns are more pronouncedly affected by moving stimuli (a moving spot of light, moving bar, edge, etc.). The majority of neuronal types encountered in the laminae of the superficial layers of the rhesus colliculus appear to belong to this class of so-called movement-sensitive neurons (Humphrey, 1968; Schiller and Koerner, 1971; Cynader and Berman, 1972; Schiller and Stryker, 1972; Goldberg and Wurtz, 1972a). In the colliculus of the squirrel monkey movement-sensitive neurons form a smaller population of neurons and in this primate such neurons appear to be localized to a deeper compartment of the superficial layers (Kadoya et al., 1971b). Neurons which respond to different wavelengths of light have been reported in the squirrel monkey (Kadoya et al., 1971c) but not in the macaque (Schiller and Malpeli, 1977).

Receptive fields of movement-sensitive neurons vary in two-dimensional shape. When tested with flashes of stationary spots of light these neurons characteristically respond following the onset and the offset of the stimulus. In some instances, inhibitory effects are obtained from area adjacent to such excitatory on–off receptive fields.

Except for neurons that respond very well to stimuli of a limited size, i.e., no larger than the excitatory part of the receptive field, specific features of the stimulus employed do not affect the responsiveness of movement-sensitive neurons. Schiller and Koerner (1971) have referred to these neurons as "event detectors," since activity recorded from them is triggered by the mere appearance of a stationary spot or by the presence of a moving stimulus in the receptive field. Similar neurons were identified by Kadoya et al. (1971b), Cynader and Berman (1972), and Goldberg and Wurtz (1972a). They have been referred to as directionally nonselective neurons (Kadoya et al., 1971b) and pandirectional neurons (Goldberg and Wurtz, 1972a) in reference to their sensitivity to any direction of stimulus movement.

Other movement-sensitive neurons referred to as directionally selective neurons respond more pronouncedly to straight moving edges aligned perpendicular to one direction (the preferred direction) of stimulus movement. Stimuli moved in the opposite direction (the null direction) have no effect or they inhibit the spontaneous activity of discharging neurons (Goldberg and Wurtz, 1972a). Though the direction of stimulus movement which is most effective in eliciting responses is usually opposite to the null direction, movements affecting the discharge rate of directionally selective neurons is not specifically limited to a single direction of movement (Kadoya et al., 1971b; Goldberg and

Wurtz, 1972a). In the squirrel monkey, one direction of stimulus movement may have an inhibitory rather than an excitatory effect (Kadoya *et al.,* 1971b).

In alert behaving monkeys, Goldberg and Wurtz (1972b) utilized saccadic eye movements as a means of displaying the attention of these animals for visual stimuli. With this device these workers were able to demonstrate a typical onset response with stationary spots of light and also augmentation or enhancement of the onset response which was associated with the production of saccadic eye movements to one and the same stimulus. These workers suggest that superficial tectal neurons may be involved in sensory or motor mechanisms that differ from those that are strictly associated with the production of eye movements per se.

2. Intermediate Layers. The receptive fields of neurons in the intermediate layers, though usually larger, are very similar to those described for superficial collicular neurons. Despite the similarities in receptive-field organization, differences in the stimulus parameters used to drive these neurons and their response properties have made it possible for several investigators (Schiller and Koerner, 1971; Schiller and Stryker, 1972; Cynader and Berman, 1972) to identify three neuronal types. These are neurons that respond to the sudden appearance of a stimulus or novel stimuli ("newness" or "novelty detectors"), neurons that are driven by quick short stimulus movements ("jerk detectors"), and neurons that are activated by one end of a long dark bar (tongue). Neurons intermediate in character to these three types and cells that are more difficult to categorize are also encountered in the intermediate and deep layers (Cynader and Berman, 1972). Typically, newness and some jerk detectors habituate to repetitive stimulation (Cynader and Berman, 1972).

In alert behaving animals the discharge of other neurons in the intermediate layers is related to saccadic (Schiller and Koerner, 1971; Wurtz and Goldberg, 1972a) or to either saccadic or smooth pursuit eye movements (Schiller and Koerner, 1971). Most eye movement neurons do not depend on orbital relationships (Schiller and Koerner, 1971; Schiller and Stryker, 1972; Wurtz and Goldberg, 1972a).

Neurons associated with saccadic eye movements have motor or eye movement fields—specific areas of the visual field to which the eyes orient following discharges. In the colliculus of one side, contralateral eye movement fields are more common than ipsilateral fields (Schiller and Koerner, 1971; Wurtz and Goldberg, 1972a). In some instances, eye movement neurons also have visual receptive fields. Though movement fields and receptive fields occupy the same area of visual space, they do not necessarily completely overlap one another (Wurtz and Goldberg, 1972a). Sensory cues in the visual field and motor responses possibly in the form of saccadic eye movements are thus brought into synaptic relationship in the intermediate layers. This may be correlated with the projection of the retina and certain areas of cortex upon the colliculus and the collicular motor map described by others.

  3. *Deep Layers.*   Except for differences in receptive-field size many neurons of the deep layers are not unlike those found in the more superficial layers (Cynader and Berman, 1972). Others, however, respond to large dark stimuli and readily habituate if the stimuli are repeatedly introduced to the field. Still others found in the deep and the intermediate layers respond with long-lasting discharges (Cynader and Berman, 1972). Eye movement neurons are also encountered in the deep gray layers, but these do not appear to possess visual receptive fields (Schiller and Koerner, 1971; Schiller and Stryker, 1972). In both intermediate and deep layers a small population of collicular neurons responds to nonvisual stimuli. Bimodal visual–tactile and visual–auditory, and trimodal visual–auditory–tactile neurons have been encountered (Cynader and Berman, 1972), but they have not been extensively studied and characterized.

C. Functional Considerations

  Various sensory and motor functions have been given to the tectal neurons described by various investigators. In the superficial layers, neurons may be involved in flux discriminations (Kadoya *et al.*, 1971b; Goldberg and Wurtz, 1972a). Movement-sensitive neurons in these layers also probably detect object motion in rather broad areas of the visual field (Goldberg and Wurtz, 1972a). Since enhanced responses occur in superficial neurons prior to eye movements, Wurtz and Goldberg (1972b) suggest that the activity is related to voluntary shifts in visual attention from one area of visual interest to another. In the deeper layers, eye movement cells may be involved in eye centering through the production of saccades, and visual tracking through smooth pursuit eye movements (Schiller and Koerner, 1971). On the other hand, collicular neurons below the stratum opticum may merely facilitate eye movements (Wurtz and Goldberg, 1972b). In the deeper layers, multimodal neurons may utilize nonvisual information for visual localizing and tracking behavior (Gordon, 1973).

IV. Behavioral Studies

Several experimental approaches have been utilized in behavioral measures of collicular function in primates. These included ablation studies to characterize behavioral deficits (Pasik *et al.*, 1966; Anderson and Symmes, 1969; Casagrande *et al.*, 1972; Wurtz and Goldberg, 1972b; Keating, 1974), stimulation studies to characterize induced motor activity (Robinson, 1972; Schiller, 1972; Schiller and Stryker, 1972), and electrophysiological recordings of cellular responses during visual activity. The results from this last approach have been discussed above.

A. Ablation Studies

Partial or total ablation of the primate colliculus was performed by Casagrande *et al.* (1972) in the tree shrew and by Pasik *et al.* (1966), Anderson and Symmes (1969), Wurtz and Goldberg (1972a,b), and Keating (1974) in the macaque. The postoperative testing procedures used by these investigators have varied greatly.

Gross behavioral patterns involving eye movements and cage behavior were studied following tectal ablations in the tree shrew by Casagrande *et al.* (1972) and in the macaque by Pasik *et al.* (1966). Casagrande and her colleagues found that tree shrews with bilateral collicular lesions confined to the superficial laminae showed normal cage behavior and normal visually guided behavior, such as ability to track a food reward, while tree shrews with total bilateral collicular ablations remained motionless in their cases as if blind. No specific mention was made by these investigators of any abnormal eye movements, but their data implied that animals with superficial lesions exhibited normal eye movements while animals with deep lesions performed fewer eye movements than normal since they appeared to be blind.

While Pasik *et al.* (1966) observed definite changes in the neurological status of their monkeys following large bilateral collicular lesions and less severe changes in animals with unilateral lesions, none of these alterations persisted beyond the immediate postoperative period.

Postoperative tests for conjugate gaze (both spontaneous and pursuit movements), eye movements associated with lid closure or head turning, optokinetic or vestibular nystagmus, and eye movements in response to auditory or somesthetic stimuli were all normal following a transitory postoperative depression of some of these functions. The interpretation of such transitory deficits is difficult and they may be a direct result of edema and surgical trauma to surrounding brain areas. None of the ablations made by Pasik and her colleagues (1966) was confined to the superficial layers of the colliculus, yet none of their monkeys, even those with almost total bilateral ablations, showed behavioral disruptions as severe as those described by Casagrande et al. (1972) for more than three days following surgery. Similar observations of transient non-specific symptoms were reported by Anderson and Symmes (1969) following bilateral colliculectomy in the monkey. It was not stated but was implied in the report by Casagrande et al. (1972) that the apparent blindness of their animals with deep collicular ablations was permanent.

It appears that the colliculus in the macaque cannot serve as a discrete center for gaze since almost total ablation of the colliculus does not result in permanent disruption of gaze. This conclusion is not surprising since stimulation of many regions of the brain other than the colliculus produces eye movements. It seems that there has been a historical bias toward identifying the colliculus as a center for the control of gaze even though sufficient evidence has accumulated to show that its influence over eye movements is not essential in primates.

Formal tests of visual discrimination also were carried out in *Tupaia* by Casagrande et al. (1972). They found that none of their animals with collicular lesions, even those with normal cage behavior, could master a test involving orientation of triangles, yet this test could be mastered by animals with totally ablated striated cortex. Animals with collicular ablations performed satisfactorily in another visual discrimination task involving orientation of stripes.

Anderson and Symmes (1969) conducted four formal behavioral tests with monkeys to determine the effects of collicular and/or cortical ablations on flicker, pattern, color, and movement discriminations. As indicated above, their observations regarding the general oculomotor functions in these animals with bilateral colliculectomy agreed with those of Pasik and Pasik (1964), but they concluded that careful examination did reveal a tendency for these animals to have fewer eye movements when they were undisturbed in their cages. However, it is difficult to rule out the possibility that this may result from an attention deficit and visual neglect rather than a depression of eye movements. The point of greatest significance resulting from the behavioral measurements by Anderson and Symmes (1969) in their animals with bilateral collicular ablations in that these animals performed satisfactorily in all tests except one, that requiring a discrimination of rate of movement. There are suggestions in the literature that there are cells in the primate colliculus which have the ability to respond differentially to varied stimulus velocities (Wurtz and Goldberg, 1972a), but these cells have not been studied in detail. Similar types of cells have not been reported for the geniculostriate system and it is tempting to speculate that this one function at least may be assigned to the superior colliculus.

The testing procedure used by Anderson and Symmes (1969) involved relatively long periods of stimulus presentation (5 S). Very short stimulus durations of 200 ms used by Keating (1974) to measure a monkey's accuracy in reaching toward a correct stimulus following bilateral colliculectomy yielded an additional interesting result. His use of stimulus durations which were shorter than the time required for the completion of a fixation saccade revealed that the animals were able to perform relatively well postoperatively if the stimulus fell within the visual field of the central part of the retina and very poorly if its position required the animal to use the peripheral part of the retina to detect the stimulus. These results appear to correlate with the lack of a direct projection of the central part of the retina to the superior colliculus (Wilson and Toyne, 1970). As long as the monkey's eye was directed toward the stimulus initially, it could use its geniculostriate system in detecting the stimulus. Still it is not clear why the monkey cannot use the geniculostriate system for peripheral detection of the stimulus also since the lateral geniculate nucleus of primates receives a projection from all parts of the retina.

Wurtz and Goldberg (1972a,b) measured saccades performed by alert, behaving monkeys before and after focal or large lesions. The monkeys had been trained to fixate a target by making a saccade; these investigators found that neither the accuracy nor the speed of these movements was altered by the lesions. But the latency of a saccade to a spot of light which fell within the receptive field of the lesioned cells was increased by 150–300 ms. This was the only persistent effect which could be observed. Wurtz and Goldberg (1972a,b) theorized that the colliculus contributes to eye movements by facilitating movements toward a certain stimulus which it specifies as meriting a shift in visual attention. Without the facilitating influence of the superior colliculus the monkey can still perform all types of eye movements as rapidly and accurately as before but its reaction time will be increased due to a decreased ability to shift attention quickly.

B. Stimulation Studies

Detailed studies of the types of eye movements produced by stimulation of collicular cells have attempted to define the executive role of the monkey superior colliculus in eye movements (Schiller, 1972; Schiller and Stryker, 1972; Robinson, 1972). Schiller and Stryker (1972) compared the type of eye movement resulting from stimulation of the abducens nucleus vs. stimulation of the deep layers of the colliculus of alert monkeys. The responses from these two locations were found to differ in several characteristics. Stimulation of the abducens nucleus produced saccades which varied with the duration and frequency (up to 600 Hz) of the stimulus and which had a latency of 10–15 ms. In contrast, stimulation of the colliculus produced saccades were unaffected by increased frequency (up to 600 Hz) or duration (up to 150 ms) of the stimulus. Beyond 150 ms stimulus duration, a second saccade of the same size and direction as the first was produced. The response latency to collicular stimulation was 20–30 ms. Similar responses could be obtained from stimulation of all layers of the colliculus, but the threshold was significantly lower in the deeper layers. Below the colliculus the threshold again increased. Stimulation of the colliculus always produced conjugate saccades which were dependent upon the location of the stimulating electrode rather than upon the position of the eye in the orbit.

Robinson (1972) also noted that the only type of movement obtained by stimulation of the colliculus in the alert monkey was a saccade. His results were similar to those obtained by Schiller and Stryker (1972) with regard to latency and effect of stimulus duration and frequency. He noted also that stimulus durations beyond 130 ms (close to the 150–ms duration cited by Schiller and Stryker, 1972) caused a second saccade equal to the first. In addition Robinson (1972) studied the effect of simultaneous stimulation of two loci in the superior colliculi. Only one saccade was produced which was a weighted mean of the two saccades which would have resulted from stimulation of each point separately.

For obvious reasons very little experimental evidence is available regarding collicular function in humans, but some tests with human commissurotomy patients have provided evidence for a brainstem contribution to human visual perception (Trevarthen, 1970). In these individuals the speech center was located in the left hemisphere which received visual stimuli by way of the geniculocorticostriate system only from the right visual field. When presented with visual stimuli in the left peripheral visual field, they were still able to verbalize certain general aspects regarding form and motion of the stimuli even when they were unable to identify the objects verbally (Trevarthen, 1970; Trevarthen and Sperry, 1973). These results suggest that in man extrageniculate visual pathways may contribute to visual perception.

V. Summary and Conclusion

A. Anatomy

The laminar organization of the collicular cortex resembles that of cerebellar and cerebral cortices and suggests an integrative functional role for this midbrain structure. The various collicular laminae may not be as closely related synaptically, however, as are the laminae in other cortices (Sprague, 1975). Afferent connections provide some basis for viewing the superior colliculus as being composed of at least two functionally distinct subnuclei, one involved chiefly with visual activities and a second involved in activities utilizing multimodal sensory input. Retinotectal and corticotectal fibers from the visual cortex provide the major afferents to the superficial layers of the colliculus, while corticotectal fibers from frontal, temporal, and parietal cortex as well as nonvisual afferents from the inferior colliculus and spinal cord project to intermediate and deep layers of the primate colliculus. Similar comparisons have been made regarding efferent projections of the collicular laminae (Harting et al., 1973; Benevento and Fallon, 1975).

B. Physiology

Several neuronal types have been identified in electrophysiological recordings of collicular neurons. Units responsive to diffuse light, stationary stimuli, or moving stimuli (movement-sensitive neurons) have been identified in the superficial layers of the colliculus. Certain movement-sensitive neurons are further distinguished by their preference for moving stimuli of a particular orientation (directionally selective neurons). Similar receptive-field properties are attributed to neurons in the intermediate layers of the colliculus though there are some differences in the required stimulus parameters. In addition, neurons which discharge in association with eye movements (eye movement neurons) have been identified. The deep layers of the colliculus have units with larger receptive fields and eye movement neurons which seem to lack receptive fields. Neurons responsive to nonvisual stimuli as well as bimodal and trimodal neurons are also located in the intermediate and deep layers.

Measurements of cellular functions have focused to a large extent on responses of superficial cells to visual stimuli, but the receptive field characteristics do not appear to suit cells primarily involved in pattern vision or in tracking movements. There appears to be sufficient evidence to conclude that the colliculus does not play an essential role in vision or visual movements. Nonetheless, its subtle influence may be of great importance in the overall ability of the animal to function efficiently in a visual world. Future work should elucidate the role of these subtle influences.

C. Behavior

Collicular ablations in the macaque result in transitory depression of behavioral responses, but persistent effects could be measured only in the ability to discriminate rates of stimulus movement (Anderson and Symmes, 1969) and in the latency of saccades in response to a stimulus (Wurtz and Goldberg, 1972a,b). Behavioral measurement of primate collicular function is complicated by the extensive development of the cerebal cortex. Functions residing in the tectum of subprimates may be shared to an unknown extent by the cerebral cortex of primates, making collicular destruction less disruptive neurologically. Alternatively the superior colliculus may function as a relay nucleus but exert limited influence over the information transmitted to cerebral cortex for further processing. The few behavioral studies described above have studied collicular function only as it relates to vision. We look forward especially to the design of appropriate tests to measure the behavioral function of the superior colliculus in activities related to other sensory modalities in addition to vision.

VI. References

Abplanalp, P. 1970. Some subcortial connections of the visual system in tree shrews and squirrels. *Brain Behav. Evol. 3:*155–168.

Abplanalp, P. 1971. The neuroanatomical organization of the visual system in the tree shrew. *Folia Primatol. 16:*1–34.

Adamuk, E. 1870. Über die Innervation der Augenbewegungen. *Zbl. Med. Wiss. 8:*65–67.

Anderson, K. V., and Symmes, D. 1969. The superior colliculus and higher visual functions in the monkey. *Brain Res. 13:*37–52.

Benevento, L. A., and Fallon, J. H. 1975. The ascending projections of the superior colliculus in the rhesus monkey (*Macaca mulatta*). *J. Comp. Neurol. 160:*339–362.

Campbell, C. B. G. 1969. The visual system of insectivores and primates. *Ann. N.Y. Acad. Sci. 167:*388–403.

Campbell, C. B. G., Jane, J. A., and Yashon, D. 1967. The retinal projections of the tree shrew and hedgehog. *Brain Res. 5:*406–418.

Campos-Ortega, J. A. 1968. Descending subcortical projections from the occipital lobe of *Galago crassicaudatus*. *Exp. Neurol. 21:*440–454.

Campos-Ortega, J. A., and Clüver, P. F. De V. 1968. The distribution of retinal fibers in *Galago crassicaudatus*. *Brain Res. 7:*487–489.

Campos-Ortega, J. A., and Glees, P. 1967a. The visual subcortical connexions in the squirrel monkey (*Saimiri sciureus*). *J. Physiol. (London) 191:*93P–95P.

Campos-Ortega, J. A., and Glees, P. 1967b. The subcortical distribution of optic fibers in *Saimiri sciureus* (squirrel monkey). *J. Comp. Neurol. 131:*131–142.

Campos-Ortega, J. A., Hayhow, W. R., and Clüver, P. F. De V. 1970. The descending projections from the cortical visual fields of *Macaca mulatta* with particular reference to the question of a cortico-lateral geniculate pathway. *Brain Behav. Evol. 3:*368–414.

Casagrande, V. A., Harting, J. K., Hall, W. C., and Diamond, I. T. 1972. Superior colliculus of the tree shrew: A structural and functional subdivision into superficial and deep layers. *Science 177:*444–447.

Cynader, M., and Berman, N. 1972. Receptive-field organization of monkey superior colliculus. *J. Neurophysiol. 35:*187–200.

Giolli, R. A., and Tigges, J. 1970. The primary optic pathways and nuclei of primates. *In* C. R. Noback and W. Montagna (eds.). *The Primate Brain*. Appleton-Century-Crofts, New York. Pp. 29–54.

Goldberg, M. E., and Wurtz, R. H. 1972a. Activity of superior colliculus in behaving monkey. I. Visual receptive fields of single neurons. *J. Neurophysiol. 35:*542–559.

Goldberg, M. E., and Wurtz, R. H. 1972b. Activity of superior colliculus in behaving monkey. II. Effects of attention on neuronal responses. *J. Neurophysiol. 35:*560–574.

Goldman, P. S., and Nauta, W. J. H. 1976. Autoradiographic demonstration of a projection for prefrontal association cortex to the superior colliculus in the rhesus monkey. *Brain Res. 116:*145–149.

Gordon, B. 1973. Receptive fields in deep layers of cat superior colliculus. *J. Neurophysiol. 36:*157–178.

Harting, J. K., and Noback, C. R. 1971. Subcortical projections from the visual cortex in the tree shrew (*Tupaia glis*). *Brain Res. 25:*21–33.

Harting, J. K., Hall, W. C., and Diamond, I. T. 1972. Evolution of the pulvinar. *Brain Behav. Evol. 6:*424–452.

Harting, J. K., Hall, W. C., Diamond, I. T., and Martin, G. F. 1973. Anterograde degeneration study of the superior colliculus in *Tupaia glis*: Evidence for a subdivision between superficial and deep layers. *J. Comp. Neurol. 148:*361–386.

Hendrickson, A., Wilson, M. E., and Toyne, M. J. 1970. The distribution of optic nerve fibers in *Macaca mulatta*. *Brain Res. 23:*425–427.

Hubel, D. H., LeVay, S., and Wiesel, T. N. 1975. Mode of termination of retinotectal fibers in macaque monkey: An autoradiographic study. *Brain Res. 96:*25–40.

Huber, G. C., and Crosby, E. C. 1933. A phylogenetic consideration of the optic tectum. *Proc. Nat. Acad. Sci. U.S.A. 19*(1):15–22.

Huber, G. C., and Crosby, E. C. 1943. A comparison of the mammalian and reptilian tecta. *J. Comp. Neurol. 78:*133–168.

Humphrey, N. K. 1968. Responses to visual stimuli of units in the superior colliculus of rats and monkeys. *Exp. Neurol. 20:*312–340.

Kaas, J. H., Harting, J. K., and Guillery, R. W. 1974. Representation of complete retina in the contralateral superior colliculus of some mammals. *Brain Res. 65:*343–346.

Kadoya, S., Massopust, L. C., Jr., and Wolin, L. R. 1971a. Striate cortex-superior colliculus projections in squirrel monkey. *Exp. Neurol. 32:*98–110.

Kadoya, S., Wolin, L. R., and Massopust, L. C. Jr., 1971b. Photically evoked unit activity in the tectum opticum of the squirrel monkey. *J. Comp. Neurol. 142:*495–508.

Kadoya, S., Wolin, L. R., Massopust, L. C. Jr., 1971c. Collicular unit responses to monochromatic stimulation in squirrel monkey. *Brain Res. 32:*251–254.

Keating, E. G. 1974. Impaired orientation after primate tectal lesions. *Brain Res. 67:*538–541.

Künzle, H., Akert, K., and Wurtz, R. H. 1976. Projection of area 8 (frontal eye field) to superior colliculus in the monkey. An autoradiographic study. *Brain Res. 117:*487–492.

Kuypers, H. G. J. M., and Lawrence, D. G. 1967. Cortical projections to the red nucleus and the brain stem in the rhesus monkey. *Brain Res. 4:*151–188.

Laemle, K. L. 1968. Retinal projections of *Tupaia glis*. *Brain Behav. Evol. 1:*473–499.

Lane, R. H., Allman, J. M., and Kaas, J. H. 1971. Representation of the visual field in the superior colliculus of the grey squirrel (*Sciurus carolinensis*) and the tree shrew (*Tupaia glis*). *Brain Res. 26:*277–292.

Lane, R. H., Allman, J. M., Kaas, J. H., and Miegin, F. M. 1973. The visuo-topic organization of the superior colliculus of the owl monkey (*Aotus trivirgatus*) and the bush baby (*Galago senegalensis*). *Brain Res. 60:*335–349.

Lund, R. D. 1969. Synaptic patterns of the superficial layers of the superior colliculus of the rat. *J. Comp. Neurol. 135:*179–208.

Lund, R. D. 1970. Structural organization of the superior colliculus and dorsal lateral geniculate body of the rat. *J. Physiol. Soc. Jap. 32:*555–556.

Lund, R. D. 1972. Synaptic patterns in the superficial layers of the superior colliculus of the monkey, *Macaca mulatta*. *Exp. Brain Res. 15:*194–211.

Lund, R. D., and Lund, J. S. 1971a. Synaptic adjustment after deafferentation of the superior colliculus of the rat. *Science 171*:804–807.

Lund, R. D., and Lund, J. S. 1971b. Modifications of synaptic patterns in the superior colliculus of the rat during development and following deafferentation. *Vision Res. 3*:281–298.

Lynch, J. C., Yin, T. C. T., Talbot, W. H., and Mountcastle, V. B. 1975. A cortical source of command signals for visually evoked saccadic movements of the eyes in the monkey. *Soc. Neurosci. 1*:59 (Abstract).

Mathers, L. H. 1971. Tectal projection to the posterior thalamus of the squirrel monkey. *Brain Res. 35*:295–298.

Mehler, W. R. 1969. Some neurological species differences—*a posteriori*. *Ann. N.Y. Acad. Sci. 167*:424–468.

Mehler, W. R., Feferman, M. E., and Nauta, W. J. H. 1960. Ascending axon degeneration following anterolateral cordotomy. An experimental study in the monkey. *Brain 83*:718–750.

Mohler, C. W., and Wurtz, R. H. 1975. A new view of visual-oculomotor integration in monkey superior colliculus. *Soc. Neurosci. 1*:231. (Abstract).

Moore, R. Y., and Goldberg, J. M. 1966. Projections of the inferior colliculus in the monkey. *Exp. Neurol. 14*:429–438.

Myers, R. E. 1963. Projections of superior colliculus in monkey. *Anat. Rec. 145*:264.

Oh, S.-Y. 1973. Zur Cytoarchitektonik der Colliculi superiores des Mittelhirns bei Cercopitheciden. *Z. Mikrosk. Anat. Forsch. 87*:410–422.

Olszewski, J., and Baxter, D. 1954. *Cytoarchitecture of the Human Brain Stem.* J. B. Lippincott, Philadelphia. 199 pp.

Pasik, P., and Pasik, T. 1964. Oculomotor functions in monkeys with lesions of the cerebrum and the superior colliculi. *In* M. B. Bender (ed.). *The Oculomotor System.* Harper and Row, New York. Pp. 40–80.

Pasik, T., Pasik, P., and Bender, M. B. 1966. The superior colliculus and eye movements. *Arch. Neurol. (Chicago) 15*:420–436.

Peele, T. L. 1942. Cytoarchitecture of individual parietal areas in the monkey (*Macaca mulatta*) and the distribution of efferent fibers. *J. Comp. Neurol. 77*:693–737.

Pierson, R. J., and Carpenter, M. B. 1974. Anatomical analysis of pupillary reflex pathways in the rhesus monkey. *J. Comp. Neurol. 158*:121–144.

Ramón y Cajal, S. 1955. *Histologie du système nerveux de l'homme et des vertébrés.* Vol. II. Consejo Superior de Investigaciones Cientifícas. Instituto Ramón y Cajal. Madrid. Pp. 174–195.

Robinson, D. A. 1972. Eye movements evoked by collicular stimulation in the adult monkey. *Vision Res. 12*:1795–1808.

Scheibel, M. E., Davies, T. L., and Scheibel, A. B. 1973. Maturation of reticular dendrites: Loss of spines and development of bundles. *Exp. Neurol. 38*:301–310.

Schiller, P. H. 1972. The role of the monkey superior colliculus in eye movement and vision. *Invest. Ophthalmol. 11*:451–460.

Schiller, P. H., and Koerner, F. 1971. Discharge characteristics of single units in superior colliculus of the alert rhesus monkey. *J. Neurophysiol. 35*:920–936.

Schiller, P. H., and Malpeli, J. G. 1977. Properties and tectal projections of monkey retinal ganglion cells. *J. Neurophysiol. 40:*428–445.

Schiller, P. H., and Stryker, M. 1972. Single-unit recording and stimulation in superior colliculus of the alert rhesus monkey. *J. Neurophysiol. 35:*915–924.

Schiller, P. H., Stryker, M., Cynader, M., and Berman, N. 1974. Response characteristics of single cells in the monkey superior colliculus following ablation or cooling of visual cortex. *J. Neurophysiol. 37:*181–194.

Schroeder, D. M., and Jane, J. A. 1971. Projections of dorsal column nuclei and spinal cord to brain stem and thalamus in the tree shrew, *Tupaia glis. J. Comp. Neurol. 142:*309–350.

Spatz, W. B., Tigges, J., and Tigges, M. 1970. Subcortical projections, cortical associations, and some intrinsic interlaminar connections of the striate cortex in the squirrel monkey (*Saimiri*). *J. Comp. Neurol. 140:*155–174.

Sprague, J. M. 1975. Mammalian tectum: Intrinsic organization, afferent inputs and integrative mechanisms. *In* Sensorimotor Function of the Midbrain Tectum. *Neurosci. Res. Programs Bull. 13*(2):204–213.

Sprague, J. M., Berlucchi, G., and Rizzolatti, G. 1973. The role of the superior colliculus and pretectum in vision and visually guided behavior. *In* R. Jung (ed.). *Handbook of Sensory Physiology,* B, Vol. VII/3. Springer, New York. Pp.27–101.

Sterling, P. 1971. Receptive fields and synaptic organization of the superficial gray layer of the cat superior colliculus. *Vision Res. Suppl. 3:*309–328.

Tigges, J., and O'steen, K. W. 1974. Termination of retinofugal fibers in squirrel monkey: A re-investigation using autoradiographic methods. *Brain Res. 79:*489–495.

Tigges, J., and Tigges, M. 1969. The accessory optic system and other fibers of the squirrel monkey. *Folia Primatol. 10:*245–262.

Tigges, J., Tigges, M., and Kalaha, C. S. 1973. Efferent connections of area 17 in *Galago. Amer. J. Phys. Anthropol. 38:*393–398.

Tigges, M., and Tigges, J. 1970. The retinofugal fibers and their terminal nuclei in *Galago crassicaudatus* (Primates). *J. Comp. Neurol. 138:*87–102.

Tigges, M., Tigges, J., Luttrel, G. L., and Frazier, C. M. 1973. Ultrastructural changes in the superficial layers of the superior colliculus in *Galago crassicaudatus* (Primates) after eye enucleation. *Z. Zellforsch. Mikrosk. Anat. 140:*291–307.

Tigges, V. J. 1966. Ein experimenteller Beitrag zum subkortikalen optischen System von *Tupaia glis. Folia Primatol. 4:*103–123.

Trevarthen, C. 1970. Experimental evidence for a brainstem contribution to visual perception in man. *Brain Behav. Evol. 3:*338–352.

Trevarthen, C., and Sperry, R. W. 1973. Perceptual unity of the ambient visual field in human commissurotomy patients. *Brain 96:*547–570.

Whitlock, D. G., and Nauta, W. J. H. 1956. Subcortical projections from the temporal neocortex in *Macaca mulatta. J. Comp. Neurol. 106:*183–212.

Williams, R. L., and Warwick, R. 1975. *Functional Neuroanatomy of Man.* W. B. Saunders, Philadelphia.

Wilson, M. E., and Toyne, M. J. 1970. Retino-tectal and cortico-tectal projections in *Macaca mulatta. Brain Res. 24:*395–406.

Wurtz, R. H., and Goldberg, M. E. 1972a. Activity of superior colliculus in behaving monkey. III. Cells discharging before eye movements. *J. Neurophysiol.* *35*:575–586.

Wurtz, R. H., and Goldberg, M. E. 1972b. Activity of superior colliculus in behaving monkey. IV. Effects of lesions on eye movements. *J. Neurophysiol.* *35*:587–596.

6

Parallel Pathways Connecting the Primate Superior Colliculus with the Posterior Vermis

An Experimental Study Using Autoradiographic and Horseradish Peroxidase Tracing Methods

JOSEPH T. WEBER AND JOHN K. HARTING

I. Introduction

Since the initial report of Snider and Stowell (1944), many studies have shown that an extensive region of the posterior vermis of the cerebellum is responsive to photic stimulation (see Fadiga and Pupilli, 1964 and Armstrong, 1974, for reviews). While the pathways over which visual

JOSEPH T. WEBER AND JOHN K. HARTING • Department of Anatomy, University of Wisconsin, Madison, Wisconsin 53706. This work was supported by Grants EY01277 and BMS76-81882. J. T. Weber is supported by NIMH Fellowship MH05601.

information reaches the posterior vermis are not well established, recent studies in our laboratory have focused upon the connections between the superior colliculus, a target of the retina in all mammals, and the inferior olivary complex, the primary source of climbing fiber input to the cerebellum (Szetágothai and Rajkovits, 1959).

In our studies we have used modern neuroanatomical tracing methods to demonstrate a direct pathway from the deep layers of the superior colliculus to a restricted cell group of the medial accessory olive, i.e., subnucleus b (Bowman and Sladek, 1974). We then analyzed the cerebellar projection of subnucleus b. Our preliminary findings show that subnucleus b projects to the posterior vermis, and in particular to lobule VII. We have therefore identified one circuit by which visual information reaches the posterior vermis (i.e., a tecto-olivo-cerebellar pathway).

Our studies also reveal that, in addition to the inferior olive, two other brainstem regions receive direct input from the superior colliculus and, in turn, project to the posterior vermis. These regions are the dorsal lateral pons and the nucleus reticularis tegmenti pontis. Thus, there exist at least three parallel channels or circuits over which visual information flowing out of the deep tectal layers can reach the posterior vermis. The results of these studies will now be presented and discussed in detail.

II. Materials and Methods

We have utilized two modern neuroanatomical tracing techniques in the present investigation. In order to define the efferent pathways of the primate superior colliculus, we injected [³H]proline and [³H]leucine into various layers and quadrants of the superior colliculus in several mature squirrel (*Saimiri sciureus*) and rhesus (*Macaca mulatta*) monkeys (see Harting, 1977). Following survival periods varying from 1 to 7 days, the monkeys were killed by perfusion with 10% formalin. The brains were subsequently blocked in the stereotaxic plane, removed, and placed in 30% sucrose formalin. The tissue was then cut on a freezing microtome at 40 μm, after which the sections were mounted on pretreated slides, coated with Kodak NTB-2 emulsion, and stored in light-tight containers at 4°C. Following exposure periods ranging from 3 to 12 weeks, the slides were developed in full-strength D-19 and lightly stained with cresyl violet (Cowan *et al.*, 1972).

For our studies of olivocerebellar connections, we injected tritiated horseradish peroxidase (Geisert, 1976) into lobule VII of the posterior vermis in two squirrel monkeys. Following survival periods of 24–48 h, the animals were killed and the tissue processed according to the autoradiographic procedures described above. The exposure periods were, however, restricted to 2–3 weeks.

III. Results

A. The Tecto-Olivary Projection in the Rhesus Monkey

Figure 1 consists of a series of line drawings that show the location of transported protein within the brainstem following an injection of [³H]leucine into the left superior colliculus (level 145) of rhesus monkey 214. In this particular experiment, the tritiated precursor was deposited primarily within the deep tectal laminae, that is, those laminae which lie ventral to the fibrous stratum opticum. Two major descending tectofugal bundles, one ipsilateral and one contralateral, can be identified within the brainstem. The contralateral pathway is called the predorsal bundle or the tectospinal tract. Axons which are destined to comprise this bundle cross within the dorsal tegmental decussation (not illustrated in Fig. 1), course in a position slightly off the midline (Fig. 1), and pass through the entire length of the brainstem. Of particular interest to the present report are the numerous labeled axons which can be seen to leave the predorsal bundle and enter the caudal portion of the inferior olivary complex (Fig. 1, levels 60 and 55). The distribution of transported protein within the inferior olive is restricted to a small portion of the medial accessory nucleus which Bowman and Sladek (1974) term the subnucleus b. Less dense label is also apparent within the corresponding region (i.e., subnucleus b) of the ipsilateral inferior olive (Fig. 1, level 60). Since the ipsilateral tectofugal bundle does not pass caudal to the pons (Fig. 1, level 145), this ipsilateral field of label most likely represents the terminals of axons which cross the midline at the level of the inferior olive. It should be emphasized that subnucleus b is the sole olivary target of the superior colliculus. The density and restricted distribution of the transported protein within subnucleus b of rhesus monkey 200 is shown in Fig. 4A.

Similar experiments in several squirrel monkeys indicate that the deep tectal layers project to the same cell group of the medial accessory

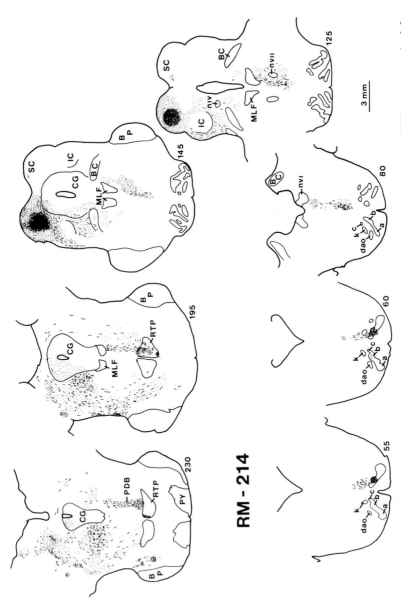

Fig. 1. The location of transported protein within the brainstem following an injection of [³H]leucine into the left superior colliculus (level 145) of rhesus monkey 214. Dashed lines indicate labeled axons, dotted regions are judged to contain terminal labels.

Figure Abbreviations

a	subnucleus a, medial accessory nucleus, inferior olive	GM	medial geniculate nucleus	NTS	nucleus tractus solitaris
b	subnucleus b, medial accessory nucleus, inferior olive	GP	gresium pontis	nIV	trochlear nerve
BC	brachium conjunctivum	IC	inferior colliculus	nVI	abducens nucleus
BP	brachium pontis	III	third ventricle	nVII	facial nerve
c	subnucleus c, medial accessory nucleus, inferior olive	k	dorsal cap of Kooy	PDB	predorsal bundle
		LR	lateral reticular nucleus	PY	pyramidal tract
CG	central gray	LRst	lateral reticular nucleus, subtrigeminal division	RTP	nucleus reticularis tegmenti pontis
CN	cochlear nucleus	MLF	medial longitudinal fasciculus	SC	superior colliculus
dao	dorsal accessory nucleus, inferior olive	NH	hypoglossal nucleus	Vi	inferior vestibular nucleus
		NP	nucleus praepositus	Vl	lateral vestibular nucleus
DR	dorsal raphe nucleus	NST	spinal nucleus of trigeminal nerve	Vm	medial vestibular nucleus
				Vs	superior vestibular nucleus

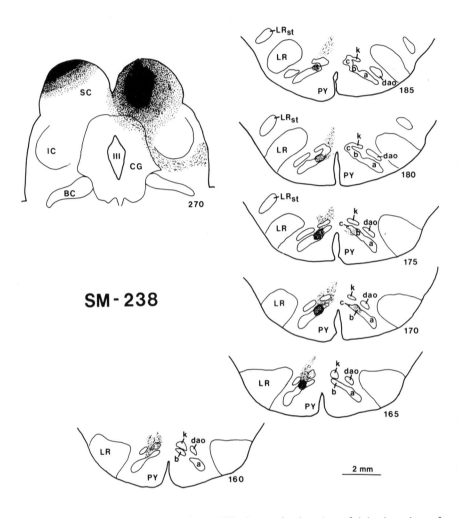

SM-238

Fig. 2. The drawing shown at level 270 shows the location of injection sites of [³H]proline within the superior colliculi of squirrel monkey 238. The injection in the left colliculus involved only the superficial layers, whereas the injection in the right invaded all tectal laminae. The remaining drawings illustrate the distribution of transported protein within the inferior olivary complex (i.e., within subnucleus b of the medial accessory olive) resulting from the injection which involved the deep layers (i.e., injection on the right). No tecto-olivary pathway could be traced from the injection which involved only the superficial layers. For abbreviations, see Fig. 1.

olive, i.e., subnucleus b. The results of one of these experiments, in which an injection was placed within each colliculus, are shown in Fig. 2. The injection of the left involved only the superficial tectal layers. No descending labeled axons could be identified arising from this particular injection. In contrast, the injection on the right invaded all tectal laminae, and numerous labeled axons could be traced into the brainstem. In particular, the contralateral subnucleus b was intensely labeled (Fig. 2). This and other experiments in squirrel monkeys establish that subnucleus b of the medial accessory olive is, as it is in rhesus monkeys, the sole target of the deep tectal laminae. The pattern of transported protein within subnucleus b of squirrel monkey 194 is shown in Fig. 4B.

Before turning to our data regarding the cerebellar target of subnucleus b, special note should be taken of another major target of the predorsal bundle, the nucleus reticularis tegmenti pontis (Fig. 1, levels 230 and 195), and of one target of the ipsilateral descending tectofugal pathway, the dorsal lateral pontine gray (Fig. 1, level 230). These two brainstem regions deserve special mention because they, like subnucleus b of the inferior olivary complex, receive input from the deep layers of the superior colliculus and, as we will subsequently show, project upon the posterior vermis. In fact, all three brainstem sites project upon the same region of the posterior vermis.

B. The Cerebellar Target of Subnucleus b

Once subnucleus b of the medial accessory olive was identified as the sole olivary target of the superior colliculus in both rhesus and squirrel monkeys, we began a series of experiments aimed at defining the region(s) of the cerebellar cortex to which it projected. Since the posterior vermis, especially lobules VI–VIII, is not only responsive to visual stimuli but also involved in eye movements (see Discussion), we felt that this particular region of the cerebellum was a likely candidate for receiving input from subnucleus b. Therefore, we injected [³H]-HRP into lobule VII of two squirrel monkeys. Since the brain was subsequently sectioned in the frontal stereotaxic plane, it was extremely difficult for us to define the injection site precisely. While the bulk of the tritiated enzyme appears to have been restricted to a small, lateral portion of lobule VII, it may have spread into the adjacent regions of lobules VI and VIII. Examination of the inferior olive revealed a dense locus of backfilled neurons only within subnucleus b of the medial

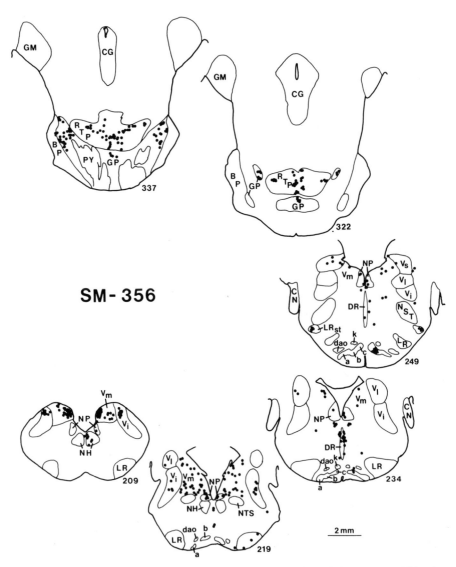

Fig. 3. The round black dots represent the location of labeled neurons within the brainstem following an injection of [³H]-HRP within lobule VII of the posterior vermis of squirrel monkey 356. For abbreviations, see Fig. 1.

accessory olive (Fig 3, level 249, and Fig. 4, C and D). While no other region of the inferior olivary complex contained backfilled neurons, several regions within the pons and medulla were moderately to heavily labeled (Fig. 3). Of particular interest was the presence of backfilled neurons within two targets of the superior colliculus, i.e., the dorsal lateral pontine gray (Fig. 3, level 337) and the nucleus reticularis tegmenti pontis (Fig. 3, levels 337 and 322). Thus, our data show that three brainstem nuclear groups, the subnucleus b of the inferior olive, the dorsal lateral pontine gray and the nucleus reticularis tegmenti pontis, receive a dense projection from the deep tectal layers of the superior colliculus and in turn project upon the same region of the posterior vermis.

IV. Discussion

In our efforts to define pathways by which visual information reaches the cerebellum, we have identified three circuits over which information flowing out of the primate superior colliculus can ultimately reach the posterior cerebellar vermis. Each of these circuits has its first order neuron within the deep tectal laminae. Second-order neurons lie within either (1) the dorsal lateral pons (tecto-ponto-cerebellar), (2) the nucleus reticularis tegmenti pontis (tecto-RTP-cerebellar), or (3) the subnucleus b of the medial accessory nucleus of the inferior olivary complex (tecto-olivo-cerebellar). Since all three circuits end within precisely the same region of the posterior vermis, visual information reaches a particular zone of the posterior vermis via both the mossy (dorsal lateral pons and the nucleus reticularis tegmenti pontis) and the climbing fiber systems (subnucleus b of the medial accessory olive).

With regard to the precise tectal origin of collicular neurons which project upon the three above-mentioned precerebellar relay nuclei, our autoradiographic studies show that they occupy a lamina (or laminae) which lies ventral to the stratum opticum. Only quite recently we have begun to analyze the specific laminar and cellular origin of each of the parallel circuits by injecting horseradish peroxidase into the inferior olive, the nucleus reticularis tegmenti pontis, and the dorsal lateral pons. Our preliminary results indicate that, at least in the cat, collicular neurons which project to the inferior olive and the dorsal lateral pons lie primarily within the intermediate tectal layers. More interestingly, we have found that cells which project to the nucleus reticularis tegmenti pontis are larger than those projecting to the inferior olivary complex.

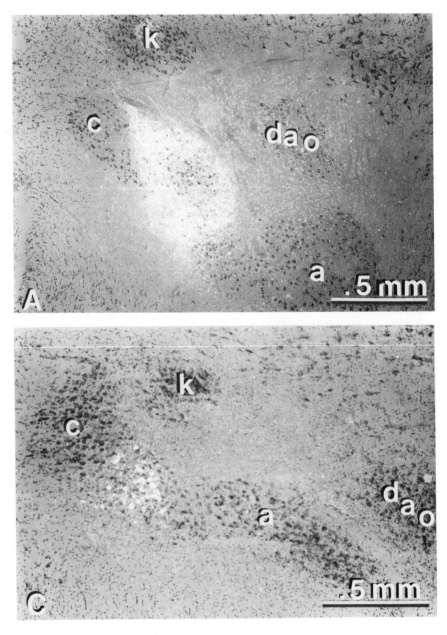

Fig. 4. (A, B) Dark-field/light-field photomicrographs showing the distribution of silver grains over subnucleus b of the medial accessory olive in rhesus monkey 200 and squirrel monkey 194, respectively, following injections of [³H]amino acids within the contralateral superior colliculus. (C) A dark-field/light-field photomicrograph showing

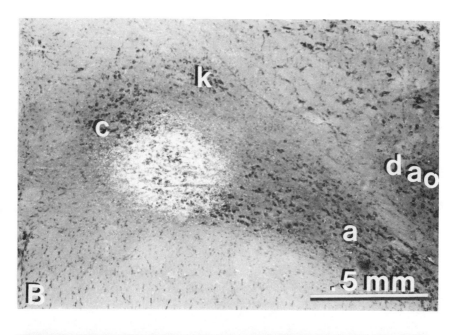

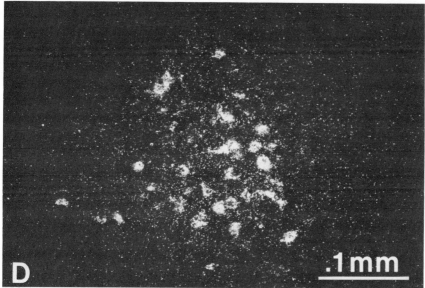

the distribution of labeled neurons within subnucleus b of the squirrel monkey following an injection of [³H]-HRP within lobule VII of the posterior vermis. (D) A dark-field photomicrograph of the labeled region shown in C.

The fact that the cells of origin of at least two of the three pathways differ morphologically suggests that they may also differ functionally.

This leads to the question of what type of visual information is being carried via the three circuits connecting the deep tectum and the posterior vermis. It is known that stimulation of cells comprising the deep tectal laminae produces contralateral saccades (Schiller and Stryker, 1972; Robinson, 1972). Deep tectal neurons also discharge prior to saccades (Schiller and Koerner, 1971; Schiller and Stryker, 1972; Wurtz and Goldberg, 1972; Robinson and Jarvis, 1974; Stryker and Schiller, 1975; Sparks, 1975; Sparks et al., 1976). Quite interestingly, stimulation of the posterior vermis also produces saccadic eye movements (Ron and Robinson, 1973), and Purkinje cells within the posterior vermis have been shown to discharge prior to saccades (Llinás, 1974). Thus, the posterior vermis and the deep tectum have certain properties which are strikingly similar. It is not surprising, therefore, that the two regions are closely interconnected.

The resemblance between the deep tectum and the posterior vermis is not limited to the similarities in their visual properties. Cells within the deep tectal layers are responsive to stimuli other than visual, that is, to auditory and somatosensory stimuli (Gordon, 1973; Dräger and Hubel, 1975; Stein et al., 1976). This finding is not unexpected since pathways which convey visual, auditory, and somatosensory information to the deep layers are well documented (Mehler et al., 1960; Steward and King, 1963; Moore and Goldberg, 1963; Garey et al., 1968; Harting, et al., 1973; Antonetty and Webster, 1975). Likewise, the posterior vermis is responsive not only to visual, but to auditory and somatosensory stimuli as well (Snider and Stowell, 1944). Thus, the three parallel pathways connecting the deep tectum and the posterior vermis are certainly sources of such multimodal information to the posterior vermal cortex.

It should be mentioned that the deep tectal layers are not the only source of visual input to the three previously discussed precerebellar relay nuclei. For example, the dorsal lateral pons, in addition to deep tectal input, receives input from the visual cortex (Nauta and Bucher, 1954; Martin, 1968; Garey et al., 1968; Campos-Ortega et al., 1970), the pretectal complex (Weber and Harting, 1975), and the ventral lateral geniculate nucleus (Graybiel, 1974). Likewise, the reticularis tegmenti pontis also receives projections from the pretectal complex (Berman, 1977). At present, visual input other than that arising from within the deep tectum has not been reported to end within subnucleus b in primates. However, studies in the opossum indicate that the olivary target of the deep tectum, which is the dorsal lateral portion of subnucleus c (Martin, personal communication) also receives input from two regions of the pontine reticular formation, the nucleus gigantocellularis and the nucleus gigantocellularis pars ventralis. These two brainstem sites receive deep tectal input (Martin, 1969). Thus, the brainstem nuclei which project upon the posterior vermis receive visual information from different sources, not just that coming from the deep tectum.

In closing, we emphasize that the posterior vermal region is not the only area of the cerebellar cortex which is considered visual. In particular, studies in the rabbit have shown that the vestibulocerebellum, i.e., the flocculus and the nodule, are also responsive to visual stimuli (Maekawa and Simpson, 1973). One of the routes by which visual input reaches the vestibulocerebellum has been well documented. This particular circuit involves a direct projection from the pretectal complex to the ipsilateral inferior olive (Mizuno *et al.*, 1973; Takeda and Maekawa, 1976). More specifically, the pretecto-olivary projection ends within the dorsal cap of Kooy and the medial and dorsal portion of the beta nucleus of the medial accessory olive. It has been reported (Alley *et al.*, 1975) that the dorsal cap of Kooy projects to both the flocculus and the nodule, while the beta nucleus projects to only the nodule. This pretecto-olivo-vestibulocerebellar pathway accounts for the physiological data which show that visual stimulation activates Purkinje cells within the vestibulocerebellum via climbing fiber afferents (Maekawa and Simpson, 1973). In addition, mossy fiber afferents to the flocculus are activated by visual stimulation (Maekawa and Takeda, 1976). Since only the lateral reticular nucleus and the perihypoglossal nuclei are sources of mossy fibers to the flocculus (Alley *et al.*, 1975), visual information has to reach these nuclei somehow. At present, no such visual pathways to these nuclei have been reported.

Acknowledgment. We thank B. Wallace for her help in all endeavors and Dr. George F. Martin for his comments on the manuscript.

V. References

Alley, K., Baker, R., and Simpson, J. I. 1975. Afferents to the vestibulo-cerebellum and the origin of the visual climbing fibers in the rabbit. *Brain Res.* 98:582–589.

Antonetty, C. M., and Webster, K. E. 1975. The organization of the spinal tectal projection. An experimental study in the rat. *J. Comp. Neurol. 163:*449–466.

Armstrong, D. M. 1974. Functional significance of connections of the inferior olive. *Physiol. Rev. 54:*358–417.

Berman, N. 1977. Connections of the pretectum in the cat. *J. Comp. Neurol. 174:*227–254.

Bowman, J. B., and Sladek, J. R. 1974. Morphology of the inferior olivary complex of the rhesus monkey (*Macaca mulatta*). *J. Comp. Neurol. 152:*299–316.

Campos-Ortega, J. A., Hayhow, W. R., and Cluver, P. F. De. 1970. The descending projections from the cortical visual fields of *Macaca mulatta* with particular reference to the question of a cortico-lateral geniculate pathway. *Brain Behav. Evol. 3:*368–414.

Cowan, W. M., Gottleib, D. I., Hendrickson, A. E., and Woolsey, T. A. 1972. The autoradiographic demonstration of axonal connections in the central nervous system. *Brain Res., 37:*21–51.

Dräger, V. C., and Hubel, D. H. 1975. Responses to visual stimulation and relationship between visual, auditory, and somatosensory inputs in mouse superior colliculus. *J. Neurophysiol. 3:*690–713.

Fadiga, A., and Pupilli, G. C. 1964. Teleceptive components of the cerebellar function. *Physiol. Rev. 44:*432–486.

Garey, L. J., Jones, E. G., and Powell, T. P. S. 1968. Interrelationships of striate and extrastriate cortex with primary relay sites of the visual pathway. *J. Neurol. Neurosurg. Psychiat. 31:*135–157.

Geisert, E. E., Jr. 1976. The use of tritiated horseradish peroxidase for defining neuronal pathways: A new application. *Brain Res. 117:*130–135.

Gordon, B. 1973. Receptive fields in deep layers of cat superior colliculus. *J. Neurophysiol. 36:*157–178.

Graybiel, A. M. 1974. Visuo-cerebellar and cerebello-visual connections involving the ventral lateral geniculate nucleus. *Exp. Br. Res. 20:*303–306.

Harting, J. K. 1977. Descending pathways from the superior colliculus: An autoradiographic analysis in the rhesus monkey (*Macaca mulatta*). *J. Comp. Neurol. 173:*583–612.

Harting, J. K., Hall, W. C., Diamond, I. T., and Martin, G. F. 1973. Anterograde degeneration study of the superior colliculus in *Tupaia glis*: Evidence for a subdivision between superficial and deep layers. *J. Comp. Neurol. 148:*361–386.

Llinás, R. 1974. Motor aspects of cerebellar control. *The Physiologist 17:*19–46.

Maekawa, K., and Simpson, J. I. 1973. Climbing fiber responses evoked in vestibulocerebellum of rabbit visual system. *J. Neurophysiol. 36:*649–666.

Maekawa, K., and Takeda, T. 1976. Electrophysiological identification of the climbing and mossy fiber pathways from the rabbit's retina to the contralateral cerebellar flocculus. *Brain Res., 109:*169–174.

Martin, G. F. 1969. Efferent tectal pathways of the opossum. *J. Comp. Neurol. 135:*209–244.

Mehler, W. R., Feferman, M. E., and Nauta, W. J. H. 1960. Ascending axon degeneration following anterolateral cordotomy. An experimental study in the monkey. *Brain 83:*718–750.

Mizuno, N., Mochizuki, K., Akimoto, C., and Matsushimi, R. 1973. Pretectal projections to the inferior olive in the rabbit. *Exp. Neurol. 39:*498–506.

Moore, R. Y., and Goldberg, J. M. 1963. Ascending projections of the inferior colliculus in the cat *J. Comp. Neurol. 121:*109–135.

Nauta, W. J. H., and Bucher, V. M. 1954. Efferent connections of the striate cortex of the albino rat. *J. Comp. Neurol. 100:*257–285.

Robinson, D. A. 1972. Eye movements evoked by colliculus stimulation in alert monkey. *Vision Res. 12:*1795–1809.

Robinson, D. L., and Jarvis, C. D. 1974. Superior colliculus neurons studies during head and eye movements of the behaving monkey. *J. Neurophysiol. 37:*533–540.

Ron, S., and Robinson, D. A. 1973. Eye movements evoked by cerebellar stimulation in the alert monkey. *J. Neurophysiol 36:*1004–1022.

Schiller, P., and Koerner, F. 1971. Discharge characteristics of single units in superior colliculus of the alert rhesus monkey. *J. Neurophysiol., 34:*920–936.

Schiller, P. H., and Stryker, M. 1972. Single unit recording and stimulation in superior colliculus of the alert rhesus monkey. *J. Neurophysiol. 35:*915–925.

Snider, R., and Stowell, A. 1944. Receiving areas of the tactile, auditory and visual systems in the cerebellum. *J. Neurophysiol. 7:*331–357.

Sparks, D. L. 1975. Response properties of eye movement-related neurons in the monkey superior colliculus. *Brain Res. 90:*147–152.

Sparks, D. L., Holland, R., and Guthrie, B. L. 1976. Size and distribution of movement fields in the monkey superior colliculus. *Brain Res. 113:*21–34.

Stein, B. E., Magelhaes-Castro, B., and Kruger, L. 1976. Relationship between visual and tactile representation in cat superior colliculus. *J. Neurophysiol. 39:*401–419.

Steward, W. A., and King, R. B. 1963. Fiber projections from the nucleus caudatus and the spinal trigeminal nucleus. *J. Comp. Neurol. 121:*271–295.

Stryker, M. P., and Schiller, P. H. 1975. Eye and head movement evoked by electrical stimulation of monkey superior colliculus *Exp. Brain Res. 23:*103–112.

Szentágothai, J., and Rajkovits, K. 1959. Über den Ursprung der Kletterfasern des Kleinhirn. *Z. Anat. Entwicklungsgesch. 121:*130–141.

Takeda, T., and Maekawa, K. 1976. The origin of the pretecto-olivary tract. A study using the horseradish peroxidase method. *Brain Res. 117:*319–325.

Weber, J. T., and Harting, J. K. 1975. On the connections of the pretectum of the tree shrew (*Tupaia glis*). *Neur. Sci. Abst. 1:*45.

Wurtz, R. H., and Goldberg, M. E. 1972. Activity of superior colliculus in behaving monkey. III. Cells discharging before eye movements. *J. Neurophysiol. 35:*575–586.

7

The Organization of Visual Cortex in Primates

Jon H. Kaas

> . . . *it is important to recognize the general concept that the cortex is by no means uniform in function and structure and is made up of a mosaic of different areas.* . . .

W. E. Le Gros Clark, 1959

I. Introduction

The purpose of this chapter is to consider how visual cortex is subdivided and interconnected in primates. Subdividing neocortex has long been a problem for neuroscientists. It has been clear that for each sensory system the cortex contains a number of interrelated parts or areas, but it has been difficult to determine the exact number, location, and interconnections of the cortical areas of a system in any mammal. Differences in histological structure were first used to subdivide neocortex, but it was difficult or impossible to determine the significance of

Jon H. Kaas • Department of Psychology, Vanderbilt University, Nashville, Tennessee 37240.

most of the areas so demarcated. Thus, Campbell (1905) parceled the neocortex of man into 20 distinct zones; Brodmann (1909) followed with 47, and C. and O. Vogt (1919) distinguished 200 fields. Later investigators postulated various numbers, with Lashley and Clark (1946) taking an extreme position and arguing that the cortex of man (or rat for that matter) contained no more than 7–10 subdivisions of functional significance. Later, considerable progress was made when the electrophysiological investigations of Woolsey, Adrian, and others established the primary and secondary sensory areas as detailed representations of sensory surfaces. More recently, microelectrode recordings have been used to determine the extent and boundaries of such sensory representations accurately and to relate these areas precisely to histological subdivisions of neocortex. In the more advanced brains, the sensory and motor areas, so clearly delimited by electrophysiological means, were found to constitute only a fraction of the total cortical surface. Much of the cortex, the so-called association cortex, was "silent" during recording and further subdivision was not possible. This condition has proven to be largely an artifact of the anesthetics popular at the time, and it is now clear that most of the cortex of higher primates responds to at least one modality. Furthermore, microelectrode recordings indicate that much of "association cortex" is subdivided into a number of separate areas, each of which contains a detailed map of a sensory surface such as the retina, skin, or cochlear partition.

As valid subdivisions of the brain have become established, it has been possible to determine how these subdivisions connect to one another by using degeneration and intraaxonal transport methods. Considerable information has now accumulated on how the visual cortex of some primates is subdivided and how these divisions are interconnected. Clearly, visual cortex in primates consists of approximately ten or more separate areas, and each of these areas appears to connect to many of the other cortical areas, as well as to a number of subcortical structures. Thus, we appear to have a system of a relatively large number of functionally distinct, but complexly interrelated parts. So far, the number, locations, internal organization, and connections of only some of these parts are known, and only for some primates. Consequently, we do not yet know the complete organization for any primate or the full extent of the possible differences from primate to primate. Nevertheless, our understanding of the organization of visual cortex in primates is far ahead of what it was only a few years ago. Some of the evidence and conclusions basic to this understanding are reviewed on the following pages.

II. The Visual Areas

A. The Traditional View of Visual Cortex

The traditional view of the organization of visual cortex of primates stems from the early architectonic studies of Brodmann (1909), Campbell (1905), and Elliot Smith (1907). In their view, a primary receiving area in the occipital lobe was bounded anteriorly by a visual psychic or association region. The association region was somewhat differently subdivided into two separate areas by Elliot Smith and Brodmann, and Brodmann's scheme of a primary area (area 17) surrounded by two concentric rings or bands of association cortex (areas 18 and 19) became standard. Later, a popular elaboration of the classical view was to consider each of the three subdivisions of visual cortex as a separate and complete representation of the contralateral visual hemifield. The initial evidence for a representation in area 17 came from clinical neurology. Since restricted lesions of area 17 were found to produce restricted scotomas, or areas of greatly impaired vision, in the half of the visual field opposite the lesion, and the region of impaired vision depended on the location of the lesion, it became apparent from clinical cases that the contralateral hemifield is systematically represented in area 17 (see Holmes, 1962). Later the details of this representation were determined by electrophysiological (Talbot and Marshall, 1941; Cowey, 1964; Allman and Kaas, 1971b; Daniel and Whitteridge, 1961) and anatomical methods (Polyak, 1957) in monkeys as well as in other mammals. The view that area 18 of primates is a second representation was in part based on recordings from cats and rabbits which suggested that the secondary area represents the visual hemifield as a "mirror image" of the primary representation. The assumption that area 18 also represents the visual field in primates has recently been supported by recording and anatomical studies, but the second representation is distinctly different from the first in visuotopic organization (see below). Finally, recordings in cats suggested that area 19 corresponds to a third systematic representation as a "mirror image" of area 18, and anatomical studies of connections have been used to support the extension of this concept to primates (Zeki, 1969, 1974; Cragg, 1969; Whitteridge, 1973). However, a considerable amount of evidence argues that "area 19" of primates is not a single architectonic field or a single representation of the hemifield. Instead, area 18 is bordered by a number of distinct visual areas (see below).

In addition to the "first three visual areas," traditional schemes of cortical organization have included infratemporal (IT) cortex as part of the visual system since the discovery of the importance of the temporal lobes in vision by Klüver and Bucy (1939). More recently studies of behavior after lesions of different parts of IT cortex suggest that IT cortex is not a single functional zone (see Mishkin, 1972), but the full extent and number of subdivisions in the IT cortex are not clear.

B. The Primary Visual Area

The primary visual area (V I) contains a topological transformation of the contralateral visual hemifield. The basic nature of the primary representation has been demonstrated by a number of procedures, but only eletrophysiological mapping methods permit a full and detailed exploration of a cortical representation. The mapping method depends on recording with microelectrodes from a large number of recording sites within an area and determining receptive fields for neurons at each site. Such information can then be used to construct a diagram of the way visual space is represented within the area. Figure 1 shows how the visual hemifield is represented in V I of the owl monkey, *Aotus*, and illustrates several features of V I that are typical of primates. First, the unfolded representation is a simple transformation of the visual hemifield in which all adjacent points in the hemifield correspond to adjacent points in the representation. This is a topological representation and has been called a first-order transformation (Allman and Kaas, 1974a). Second, it is apparent that much of the area relates to central vision. Since the owl monkey is a nocturnal primate, this second feature is even more pronounced in most other primates. As a result of the expanded representation of central vision, most of the outer border of V I corresponds to the zero vertical meridian, i.e., a vertical line through the center of gaze corresponding to the line of decussation of the retina. The zero horizontal meridian passes across the middle of the area dividing it into halves corresponding to the upper and lower quadrants of the

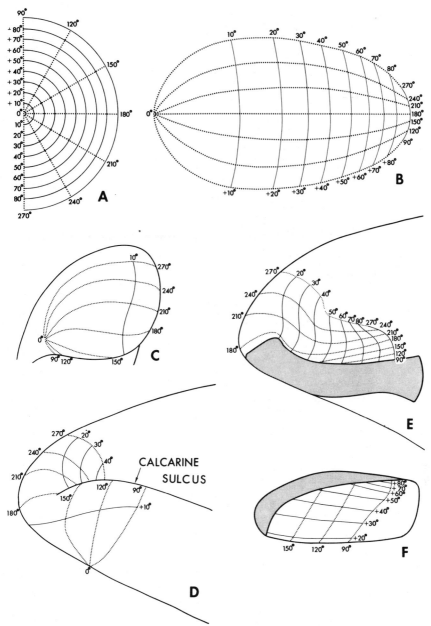

Fig. 1. The representation of the visual hemifield in V I of the owl monkey. A. A perimeter chart of the visual hemifield. B. The unfolded topological distortion of the representation of the hemifield in V I. C–F: Views of the occipital lobe in stages of dissection showing the organization of V I. C, posterior view; D, medial view; E, medial view with the lower bank of the calcarine fissure removed; F, the lower bank of the calcarine fissure viewed dorsally. (From Allman and Kaas, 1971b.)

opposite hemifield. Small electrolytic lesions made at the border of V I during recording experiments indicate that the primary representation is coextensive with the architectonically very distinctive striate cortex or area 17 of Brodmann (1909).

C. The Secondary Visual Area

Evidence of a second systematic representation of the visual field adjacent to striate cortex was first discovered by Talbot (1941) in electrophysiological mapping experiments on the cat, and later termed V II by Woolsey and Fairman (1946). In primates, the second visual area occupies a long narrow belt of tissue surrounding most of V I. The representation of the visual field is a different type in V II, and the primary and secondary visual areas are interconnected in a manner suggesting that they function together as a higher-order unit.

Insofar as is known, V II in all mammals borders the portion of V I that represents the zero vertical meridian and the representation of this line forms the common border between the two areas. Since the portion of the complete border of V I formed by the vertical meridian varies from species to species with the extent of the expansion of the representation of retina along the line of decussation, the portion of V I bordered by V II also varies. In all primates, central vision at the intersection of the horizontal and vertical meridians is greatly expanded in the cortical representations with the result that the vertical meridian forms most of the outer border of V I. Even in nocturnal primates such as the owl monkey which depend less on central vision, V II borders as much as 90% of V I, and this proportion assuredly is higher in diurnal primates. By stretching around most of V I, the second visual area becomes a long narrow belt in primates.

One way V II can become an elongated belt and still represent the hemifield without extreme distortions is to "split" and no longer maintain a simple topological organization. V I is a simple topological representation in that adjacent loci in the contralateral half of the visual field are *always* represented in adjacent cortical loci. However in V II of prosimians (Allman and Kaas, unpublished), New World monkeys (Allman and Kaas, 1974a; Spatz *et al.*, 1970), Old World monkeys (Cragg, 1969; Zeki, 1969, 1974), and probably other primates, the representation of the horizontal meridian splits beyond the central few degrees of vision and forms most of the anterior border of V II (Fig. 2).

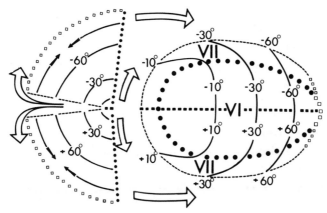

Fig. 2.   V II as a split or second-order transformation of the visual hemifield. The hemifield (left) is split and distorted (right) to surround most of V I. Dots mark the vertical meridian; filled squares and dashes, the horizontal meridian; open squares, the temporal periphery.

Thus, except for the central few degrees, the upper and lower quadrants of the visual field are represented in the lateral and medial wings of the V II belt, respectively. For paracentral and peripheral vision, adjoining parts of the visual field on each side of the horizontal meridian are represented in quite distant parts of V II. Allman and Kaas (1974a) have referred to the topological representation of V I as a first-order transformation and the split representation of V II as a second-order transformation of the visual field. Both types of representation are found in other areas of visual cortex.

The long common border of V I with V II resulting in the elongation of V II and the split in the representation in V II suggests that it is important for any part of V II representing any given location of the hemifield to be located close to the part of V I representing the same location. It is known, in fact, from fiber degeneration studies (Tigges *et al.*, 1973a) that homotopic points in V I and V II are interconnected. The relationship of V II to V I allows these connections to be over relatively short pathways. Allman and Kaas (1974a) have suggested that one of the functions of V II is to process information relayed from V I further and then feed back to modulate the output of V I. Viewed in this perspective, V II can be considered to function as an *adjunct* to VI.

The second visual area can be identified with a distinct architectonic zone that probably should be termed area 18 after Brodmann

(1909). It is clear that in a number of mammals, V II corresponds to area 18 as described and delimited by Brodmann. Electrophysiological mapping studies (Allman and Kaas, 1971b, 1974a, and unpublished; Cowey, 1964) and studies of the projections of V I onto V II (Spatz *et al.*, 1970; Tigges *et al.*, 1973) show a close correspondence between V II and area 18 as defined in prosimians and New World monkeys (Le Gros Clark, 1931; Solnitzky and Harman, 1946; Brodmann, 1909). However, the distinctiveness of area 18 varies considerably from species to species, and Brodmann appears to have included parts of adjoining cortex in "area 18" of Old World monkeys. Detailed electrophysiological maps of V II of Old World monkeys are not available, but recordings from V II (Allman and Kaas, unpublished) and the pattern of projections from V I (Kuypers *et al.*, 1965; Zeki, 1969; Cragg, 1969) in rhesus monkeys indicate that only the posterior third or so of the classically defined area 18 belt actually relates to V II. Thus, the designated architectonic belt is much too wide for V II in Old World monkeys. In order to have an architectonic label that applies to the homologous area across species, it appears useful to redefine area 18 in those species where the classically defined "area 18" is at variance with V II.

D. Visual Areas beyond V II

Visual areas I and II have been demonstrated in a broad range of mammals, including several primates, and it is quite reasonable to suppose that these areas exist in all primates. A problem in discussing other visual areas is that no other visual areas have been clearly identified in several mammalian orders, or even in many primates. A wide band of cortex just anterior to V II has been identified as visual in prosimians, New World monkeys, and Old World monkeys from recordings of neurons activated by visual stimuli and from anatomical demonstrations of projections from the primary and secondary visual areas, but the internal organization and even the full extent of this band are not well established in any primate. As noted, the cortex bordering the anterior margin of area 18 was considered to be a single functional area, area 19, by Brodmann, but a few other investigators concluded that the cortex anterior to area 18 is not uniform in structure in at least some primates. For example, in the brains of prosimians, where the anterior border of area 18 is relatively easy to define architectonically, Solnitzky and Harman (1946) restricted "area 19" to a small portion of the border of area 18 on the dorsomedial surface of the cerebral hemisphere, while Le Gros Clark (1931) was unable to identify an area 19 and described several histological subdivisions bordering area 18.

In the owl monkey it has been possible to subdivide some of the visually responsive cortex ahead of V II into several separate areas of the visual field on the basis of both electrophysiological mapping studies and histological structure. Collectively, these additional visual areas have been called the third tier, with V I and V II making up the first two tiers (Allman and Kaas, 1975). The third tier areas include much of the cortex defined by Brodmann as area 19, but this clearly does not form a single representation of the visual field and is not uniform in histological structure. Some of the additional visual areas identified in the owl monkey (see Figs. 3 and 4) appear to exist in other primates, but it is quite possible that the third tier and other visual association cortex are organized, in part, differently in various primates with some areas present in all primates and others existing in only some primate lines. The following description of visual areas rostral to V II is based largely on the owl monkey since more is known about the organization of visual association cortex in this New World monkey than for any other primate.

1. The Middle Temporal Visual Area. A portion of the temporal lobe of the owl monkey represents the visual hemifield as a first-order transformation. This representation has been called the middle temporal visual area (MT) by Allman and Kaas (1971a). In organization, MT is a smaller version of V I. As in V I, the representation of the zero vertical meridian forms most of the outer border of MT, and the horizontal meridian divides MT into adjoining halves of approximately the same size corresponding to the upper and lower visual quadrants. Also like V I, MT is easy to identify histologically. As in primary sensory areas, the cells in layers IV and VI of MT are densely packed, and the area is heavily myelinated with prominent inner and outer bands of Baillarger. MT stands out in strong contrast to adjoining cortex even in fresh brain sections by the whiteness of the myelinated nerve fibers. This distinction is even more obvious after fiber stains for myelin. One advantage of this architectonic distinctiveness is that MT can be identified in experimental material, and it has thus been possible to confirm the location of lesions and injections in MT.

By electrophysiological mapping methods, MT has been identified in only one other primate, the prosimian *Galago* (Allman *et al.,* 1973). However, on the basis of location, myeloarchitecture, and connections,

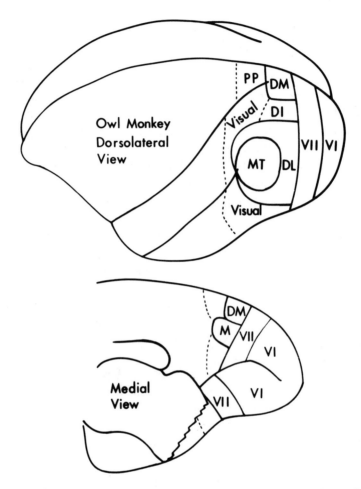

Fig. 3.   The visual areas of the owl monkey. V I, the primary visual area; V II, the secondary visual area; DI, dorsointermediate area; DL, dorsolateral area; DM, dorsomedial area; M, medial area; MT, middle temporal area; PP, posterior parietal area. The region marked visual (dashed lines) contains additional representations that have not yet been mapped in detail. The medial view is reversed.

MT has been identified in other New World monkeys such as the squirrel monkey (Spatz, *et al.,* 1970) and the marmoset (Spatz and Tigges, 1972, 1973). In addition, recordings from the temporal cortex of the slow loris, another prosimian, are consistent with the concept of MT (Krishnamurti *et al.,* unpublished). There is less information about this region in Old World monkeys and higher primates. The pattern of projections from striate cortex in rhesus monkeys to the posterior bank of the superior temporal sulcus (Kuypers *et al.,* 1965; Cragg, 1969; Zeki, 1969) strongly suggests the presence of MT, but further studies of organization, architectonics, and connections would be useful in establishing homologies, as well as the exact location and full extent of the area.

2. *The Dorsolateral Crescent.* In the owl monkey, another representation of the contralateral hemifield is found in a histologically distinct crescent-shaped area which wraps around most of MT. This representation has been called the dorsolateral visual area (DL) (Allman and Kaas, 1974b). Within DL, the representation of the hemifield is a second-order transformation like V II, and the relationship of DL to MT appears to be similar to the V II–V I relationship. DL and MT have a common border along the representation of the vertical meridian. The representation of all but the central part of the

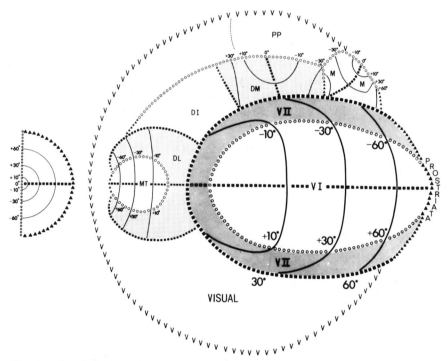

Fig. 4. A schematic unfolding of visual cortex of the owl monkey showing the visuotopic organization of some of the visual areas. Reference coordinates are on the perimeter chart on the left. Abbreviations are as in Fig. 3. (From Allman and Kaas, 1976.)

horizontal meridian in DL is split, so that DL wraps around MT with the outer boundary of DL formed by the horizontal meridian. The representation of the lower quadrant in DL adjoins the lower quadrant of MT, and the upper quadrant of DL adjoins the upper quadrant of MT. If a lesion is made in MT so that cortex on each side of the horizontal meridian is damaged, projections to separate locations in the medial and lateral wings of the DL crescent are revealed (Spatz and Tigges, 1972), as would be expected from projections from a first- to second-order transformation. It is not known if the crescent projects back to MT, but in terms of related visuotopic organizations and connections from MT, the crescent and MT together form a miniature mirror image of the V I-V II system. Thus, the anatomical relationships suggest that DL and MT as well as V II and V I form functional pairs or higher-order units of the visual system.

It is not certain if DL is organized in the same way or even exists in other primates. The pattern of connections from V II suggests the presence of a somewhat larger DL in squirrel monkeys (Tigges *et al.*, 1974). Incomplete electrophysiological mapping studies in galagos indicate DL or a DL-like area between V II and MT (Allman and Kaas, unpublished). In rhesus monkeys, the pattern of connections from V II (Zeki, 1971) is consistent with the concept of DL, but the total pattern of corticocortical connections suggests further complexities including, perhaps, additional visual areas.

3. The Dorsomedial Area.   Another systematic representation of the contralateral hemifield that has been identified in owl monkeys has been termed the dorsomedial visual area (DM) (Allman and Kaas, 1975). The area is located on the dorsal and medial surfaces of the occipital lobe in densely myelinated cortex just anterior to V II. Within the representation, the upper and lower quadrants are partially separated as the horizontal meridian splits in peripheral vision to form much of the outer boundary of DM. Thus, DM is a second-order transformation like V II and DL. However, unlike V II and DL, the split in DM does not result in a spatially contiguous relationship along the vertical meridian with a first-order representation. Instead, the split allows some of DM border along the horizontal meridian to border the horizontal meridian of V II. The reasons for this arrangement may be primarily developmental rather than functional, since there are no major interconnections between V II and DM (Wagor *et al.*, 1975).

The DM has not yet been identified in other primates. However, projections from MT to the expected location of DM just anterior to

V II in the squirrel monkey (Spatz and Tigges, 1972) suggest that DM may exist in this New World monkey. In two prosimians, the bush baby (Allman and Kaas, unpublished experiments) and the slow loris (Krishnamurti *et al.*, unpublished experiments), some of the dorsal cortex near the medial wall just anterior to V II responds to stimuli in the upper visual quadrant. These findings suggest, but do not demonstrate, DM.

4. The Medial Area. A visual area (M) on the medial wall of the cerebral hemisphere of the owl monkey just anterior to V II is unusual in that the representation of central vision is not greatly expanded as in all other known visual areas (Allman and Kaas, 1976). In striate cortex, for example, about 30% of the area is devoted to the central 10° of vision, while in M only about 5% of the area represents the central 10°. Presumably, M is specialized for visual functions related to paracentral and peripheral vision. M is a second-order transformation with the horizontal meridian partially split to form part of the border with V II along the horizontal meridian and part of the border with DM along the horizontal meridian. Projections to the presumed location of M from other subdivisions of visual cortex (Spatz and Tigges, 1972; Martinez-Millán and Holländer, 1975) suggest the existence of M in other New World monkeys, but M has not been clearly demonstrated in other primates.

5. Other Visual Areas. For several other regions of visually responsive cortex in the owl monkey there is evidence of separate and distinct visual areas, but the electrophysiological mapping of these regions is incomplete (Allman and Kaas, unpublished). One of these regions is in the posterior parietal cortex just medial to the end of the Sylvian sulcus. This cortex, the posterior parietal area, is interesting in that it may be a center for integrating visual and somatosensory information. Neurons in the posterior parietal area have large receptive fields and appear to form a systematic organization, although the details of this organization are not yet clear. The area receives input from other subdivisions of visual association cortex and may receive input from somatosensory association cortex as well. The posterior parietal area is part of the cortex Brodmann termed area 7 in New World monkeys, and area 7 in the rhesus monkey receives input from the more anterior somatosensory association cortex, i.e., area 5 (Jones and Powell, 1970). Recordings from area 7 in rhesus monkeys are intriguing in that neurons are activated by both somatic and visual stimuli (Hyvärinen and Poranen, 1974; Mountcastle, 1975).

Another incompletely explored region is the dorsointermediate area (DI) located between DL and DM. Often it has been difficult to obtain many recordings from DI, but the area appears to represent the visual field with the lower quadrant lateral and the upper quadrant medial. Much of the outer border of DI relates to the horizontal meridian. Other recordings indicate the visual field is represented in cortex just anterior to V II on the lateral aspect of the ventral surface of the occipital lobe. The map is as yet incomplete, but this ventrolateral area represents both the upper and lower quadrants in cortex adjoining the upper quadrant representation in V II.

Cortex ventral to MT and DL in the temporal lobe of the owl monkey is also responsive to visual stimuli, and this is cortex in the position of the inferotemporal (IT) cortex of rhesus monkeys. The finding that lesions in different parts of IT cortex produce different behavioral impairments (Mishkin, 1972) suggests that this region is not a single visual area. In addition, on the basis of location it appears that the superior and posterior aspect of the IT cortex of rhesus monkeys may include parts of DL and MT. Neurons in at least part of IT have receptive fields that are involved in central vision (Gross, 1973), and at least some of the visually responsive cortex ventral to DL in the temporal lobe of owl monkeys is activated by stimuli in the center of gaze.

III. Connections

Considerable progress has been made in determining the connections of subdivisions of visual cortex by tracing degenerating axons after lesions, by tracing labeled axons after intraaxonal transport of radioactive proteins, and by the labeling of cell bodies after retrograde transport of horseradish peroxidase from axon terminals. A basic problem, however, is to clearly identify the subdivisions of cortex containing the lesion or injection site. Some areas of visual cortex are easy to identify architectonically; others are not. Investigators have naturally tended to trace projections from those subdivisions that are easy to identify. Even where the subdivision containing the lesion or injection site can be clearly identified, cortical subdivisions in which the connections terminate may not be so clearly identified. Often it is only possible to say that the projections are in the expected location of an area. A further difficulty is that cortical areas may have been defined in one primate species and connections in another, so that conclusions assume basic similarities in the positions of areas. As a result of these problems, some connections of the visual system are well established, others appear reasonable or valid but remain in doubt, and others have yet to be demonstrated.

A. Receiving and Projecting Neurons

Neocortex is stratified into layers of different cell distributions and types. The relation of intrinsic and extrinsic connections to laminar organization is better known for area 17 than for other subdivisions of visual cortex.

The connections of the layers of area 17 are shown in Fig. 5. The input from the dorsal lateral geniculate nucleus is mainly to layer IV (Hubel and Wiesel, 1972). The projections from the parvocellular layers of the lateral geniculate nucleus terminate in the lower half of layer IV, and the magnocellular layers terminate in the upper half. The parvocellular layers of the lateral geniculate nucleus also contribute to layers IIIb and I. Other input to layer I of area 17 is from area 18 (Tigges et al., 1974). Within area 17, axons from the granular cells in layers IV and IIIb relay information in a vertical manner to other cortical layers (Lund and Boothe, 1975), and the external layers project densely into layer V (Spatz et al., 1970; Martinez-Millán and Holländer, 1975). In addition, pyramidal cells in layers IIIc and V have apical dendrites gathering information from more external layers including layer I. These pyramidal cells are the principal source of efferents from area 17. Some of the IIIc pyramids project to MT (Spatz, 1975), while others apparently project to area 18 (Spatz et al., 1970). The large Meynert cells of layer V also project to MT (Spatz, 1975), while other pyramidal cells of layer V project to the superior colliculus and inferior pulvinar (Lund et al., 1975) and, presumably, other brainstem structures. Cells in layer VI project to the lateral geniculate nucleus (Lund et al., 1975).

In striate cortex of rhesus monkeys, some vertical arrangements of cells are predominately activated by one eye, other vertical arrangements by the other eye. The locations and shapes of the input related to the vertical ocular dominance columns (actually bands) have been demonstrated by anatomical methods (Hubel and Wiesel, 1972; Wiesel et al., 1974; LeVay et al., 1975). Input from one eye (via the lateral

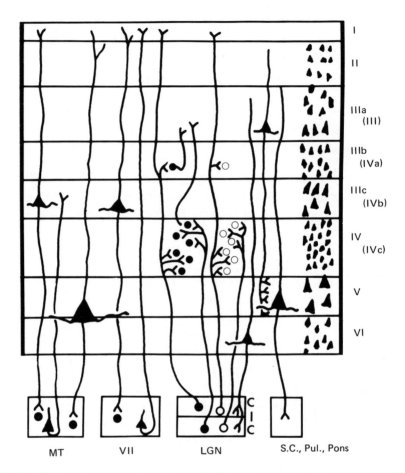

Fig. 5. The laminar connections of area 17. The diagram is based on reports on New and Old World monkeys described in the text. The major input from the parvocellular and magnocellular layers of the lateral geniculate nucleus (LGN) is divided into alternating strips or bands of tissue related to the contralateral (solid neurons) or ipsilateral (outlined neurons) eye in the rhesus monkey. Other connections are with: the middle temporal visual area, MT; the second visual area, V II; the superior colliculus, SC; the pulvinar complex, Pul; and the pons. The arrangement of cell bodies in area 17 is diagramed on the right. Two alternative schemes for numbering layers are shown. In area 17 of primates, part of what appears to be within layer III is well developed in comparison with other areas of cortex and with most other mammals and was considered part of layer IV by Brodmann. Many authors continue to follow Brodmann's designations for layers in area 17 of primates, but others have corrected for what seems to be an inconsistency and have used Brodmann's numbers in a scheme compatible with the use of these numbers in other mammals and in other cortical areas. Brodmann's layers IVa and IVb correspond to IIIb and IIIc of the corrected scheme, which is used here.

geniculate nucleus) is segregated in narrow strips of cortex that alternate with narrow strips with input from the other eye (Fig. 5). It is interesting that the strips cross the horizontal meridian in the part of striate cortex representing central vision but not in the part representing paracentral and peripheral vision. Perhaps this is related to the projection pattern from V I and V II where the projection is topographic for central vision but split at the horizontal meridian for the rest of the representation (see Fig. 2). Such distinct and separate bands related to ocular dominance do not exist in all primates. They are not present in the primitive primate (or close relative of primates) the tree shrew, where input related to each eye forms horizontal sheets rather than discontinuous bands (Casagrande and Harting, 1975; Hubel, 1975), and they are not present in the owl monkey (Kaas, et al., 1976).

The relation of connections to laminar organization seen in area 17 generally applies to other areas. Major inputs are concentrated in layer IV, although other layers including I are involved (Wagor et al., 1975; Spatz and Tigges, 1972). Outer layers relay to layer V, which appears to be the major source of efferents to subcortical structures.

B. Ipsilateral Connections

1. Area 17. Because area 17 or striate cortex can be identified with absolute certainty in primates, many investigators have placed lesions or injections in this subdivision. Each small region or point in area 17 projects to the part of area 18 representing the same visual space, insofar as can be judged by comparing electrophysiological maps of the two areas. Since V II is a representation split along the horizontal meridian, lesions in the horizontal meridian of V I result in two separate foci of degeneration in V II (Spatz et al., 1970). The connections of area 17 with area 18 are reciprocal (Tigges et al., 1973a), and points representing the same space in both areas are interconnected so that the output from area 17 is subject to feedback and modification from area 18.

A second major projection field of area 17 is MT. Projections to MT have been demonstrated in prosimians (Tigges et al., 1973b) and New World monkeys (Spatz et al., 1970) and to the probable homologue of MT in Old World monkeys (Kuypers et al., 1965; Zeki, 1969; Cragg, 1969). The projections to MT from area 17 appear to connect corresponding points in the two representations of the visual field (Spatz, 1977). MT projects back to V I (Spatz and Tigges, 1972), but it is not yet certain if this feedback interconnects homotopic points in MT and V I.

Finally, it has been argued that area 17 of rhesus monkeys connects in a point-to-point fashion to "area 19" in a manner demonstrating a systematic representation of the visual field, i.e., V III (Zeki, 1969; Cragg, 1969). The evidence for "area 19" as V III is inconclusive since the projections of only a limited part of area 17 of rhesus monkey have been determined, and these connections could be to one or more visual areas such as the third tier areas of the owl monkey. In the New World monkeys, lesions of the part of area 17 representing central vision did not produce degeneration in any other cortical areas bordering area 18 (Spatz and Tigges, 1972). However, after lesions in paracentral parts of area 17, a projection was shown to the cortex just anterior to area 18 on the medial wall of the cerebral hemisphere (Martinez-Millán and Holländer, 1975). The region of this projection field is in the expected location of M (Fig. 3). Since M has a very limited representation of central vision, this may account for the sparsity or lack of connections with central striate cortex. In any case, it appears that for both Old and New World monkeys, area 17 projects to some of the cortex bordering area 18, as well as to area 18 and MT.

2. Area 18.   Fewer studies have considered the connections of area 18 (Zeki, 1971; Tigges *et al.,* 1974; Kaas and Lin, 1977). The rostral border of area 18 is difficult to determine in New and Old World monkeys, but the approximate width of the area can be estimated from experimental studies, and lesions or injections can thereby be localized in area 18 with assurance. In addition to projecting back to area 17, at least part of area 18 projects to the region of (DL) in a manner suggesting the connection of homotopic points in the two representations. Another projection from area 18 is to DM. However, DM does not appear to project back to area 18 (Wagor *et al.,* 1975).

3. The Middle Temporal Area.   A third area that is easy to delimit is MT, which is distinguished in serial brain sections by heavy myelination. The projections of MT are shown in Fig. 6, where a lesion in MT produced a total of nine cortical foci of terminal axon degeneration (Spatz and Tigges, 1972). Since this lesion in the middle of MT necessarily involved the horizontal meridian, the foci of degeneration just above and just below MT correspond to the split or double representation of the horizontal meridian in DL. It seems probable that

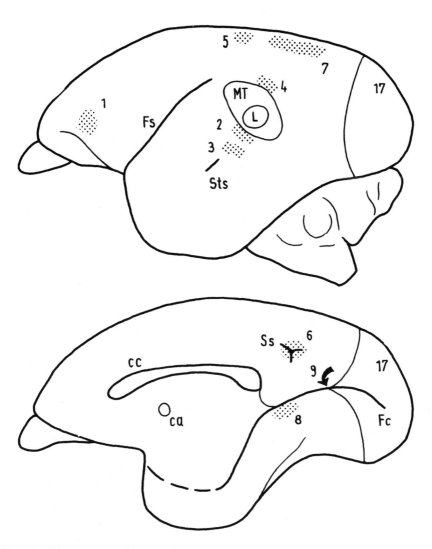

Fig. 6. The cortical efferents of the middle temporal visual area (MT) in the marmoset. A lesion (L) in MT resulted in 9 foci of terminal degeneration (stippled areas 1–9). Focus 9 (arrow) is hidden in the calcarine fissure. The medial view has been reversed. Ca, anterior commissure; CC, corpus callosum; Fc, calcarine fissure; Fs, Sylvian fissure; Ss, subparietal sulcus; Sts, superior temporal sulcus. (From Spatz and Tigges, 1972.)

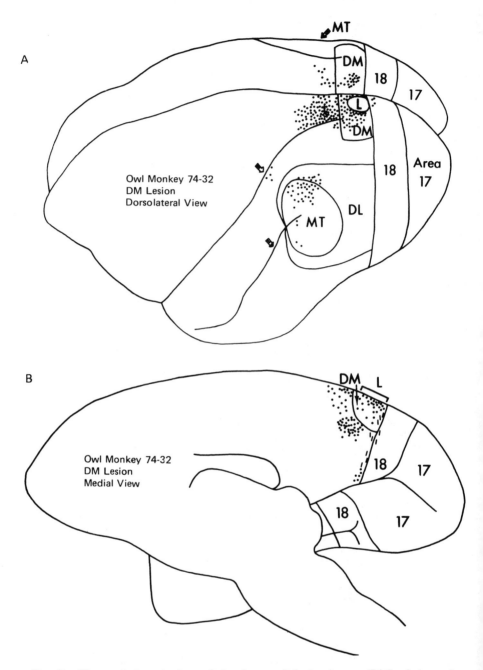

Fig. 7. The cortical projections of the dorsomedial visual area (DM) of the owl monkey. A lesion (L) results in terminal degeneration (dots) in posterior parietal cortex, the middle temporal visual area (MT), the dorsolateral crescent (DL), and cortex of the medial wall. An arrow shows the location of contralateral degeneration in MT. The medial view is reversed. (From Wagor *et al.,* 1975.)

the connections of MT with DL are between homotopic points and are reciprocal, but the projections of DL have not yet been established. Other projections of MT are to the region of DM (focus 7), the region of the posterior parietal area (focus 5), and the region of M (focus 6). Note also projections to the frontal eye fields (focus 1), to tentorial cortex just anterior to area 18 (focus 8), to IT cortex in the temporal lobe (focus 3), and to area 17 (focus 9).

4. *The dorsomedial area* is somewhat less densely myelinated than MT, but DM can also be clearly localized in experimental material. Fields of terminal degeneration after a lesion of DM are shown in Fig. 7. The major cortical output of DM is to the posterior parietal cortex just anterior to DM. In turn, posterior parietal cortex projects back to DM, as well as to several other regions of visual association cortex (Kaas *et al.,* 1977). Other connections of DM are to MT, DL, the region of M, and cortex on the anterior border of area 18 just above the calcarine fissure. This last projection field of DM suggests an additional visual area not included in Fig. 3.

5. *Subcortical projections* from area 17 (Spatz *et al.,* 1970; Hollander, 1974; Campos-Ortega and Hayhow, 1972; Spatz and Erdmann, 1974), area 18 (Lin and Kaas, 1977), MT (Spatz and Tigges, 1973), and DM (Norden *et al.,* 1978) have been determined. All these areas connect with subdivisions of the brainstem considered primarily visual in function. All project to the superior colliculus with terminations deeper in the structure than the retinal input. Some connections are reciprocal so that area 17 receives input from the dorsal lateral geniculate nucleus and the geniculate, in turn, gets a projection back from area 17. In a similar manner, MT projects to the inferior pulvinar, and the inferior pulvinar projects back to MT. The visual areas mentioned above also project to the inferior pulvinar (Lin and Kaas, 1975) and other parts of the pulvinar complex. Other subcortical projections include the pregeniculate nucleus, parts of the lateral posterior complex, the pretectum, the corpus striatum, and parts of the pons.

C. Callosal Connections

The visual representations in each cerebral hemisphere are of the opposite hemifield, and callosal connections connect the two separate halves of each representation. The interhemispheric connections are of three main types. One type relates only to the vertical meridian and serves to unify two halves into a complete field representation. The functions of connections of this type are probably like those of shorter connections within areas where neurons representing adjacent parts of visual space relate to each other over short intrinsic pathways. However, at the margin of an area where the vertical meridian is represented, long transcallosal pathways are required to connect neurons representing adjacent space on each side of the vertical meridian. A second type of interconnection relates mirror-image parts of the two hemifields. This second type of connection could function in the transfer of learned responses to stimuli in one hemifield to those stimuli in the other hemifield. A third type of callosal connection is from one visual area to several other visual areas of the opposite cerebral hemisphere. This third type presumably functions to integrate the activity of several areas in the two hemispheres.

The vertical meridian type of interconnections are most often considered in discussions of forebrain commissures. The prime example is the pathway from the 17–18 border region of one hemisphere to the 17–18 border region of the other hemisphere (Myers, 1965; Cragg, 1969; Zeki, 1970). At least some of these connecting axons are from large- and medium-sized pyramidal cells of layer III of area 18 (Glickstein and Whitteridge, 1976; Wong-Riley, 1974; Shoumura et al., 1975). The axons from these cells terminate at the posterior margin of area 18 of the opposite side, and area 17 appears to lack direct interhemispheric connections. It is possible that many or all of the subdivisions of visual association cortex have the vertical meridian type of interconnections, but such pathways would be difficult to demonstrate in small areas where it would be hard to confine lesions or injections to the representation of the vertical meridian.

Lesions or injections centered within areas away from the representation vertical meridian have been used to demonstrate symmetrical connections unrelated to the vertical meridian. Such connections are sparse or absent in area 18, but they are substantial in MT (Spatz and Tigges, 1972; Lin and Kaas, unpublished) and DM (Wagor et al., 1975). In addition, area 18, MT, DM, and posterior parietal cortex have been shown to connect asymmetrically to more than one visual area of the opposite hemisphere. Besides having the vertical meridian connections at the 17–18 border, area 18 projects transcallosally to the cortex in the region of the 18–DL border (probably DL), and to MT (Tigges et al., 1974). MT projects contralaterally to

DL as well as to MT (Spatz and Tigges, 1972), and DM projects callosally to MT and to posterior parietal cortex as well as to DM (Wagor et al., 1975). Callosal connections of posterior parietal cortex are to more than one location in the parietal cortex of the opposite hemisphere (Kaas et al., 1977). Thus, callosal connections to more than one area are common.

Since the transcallosal connections of the 17–18 border region so obviously relate to the vertical meridian, it is sometimes assumed that callosal connections in general indicate cortex where the vertical meridian is represented. However, such schemes based on callosal connections are questionable because of the other two types of connections, the mirror symmetrical callosal connections and the asymmetrical callosal connections to more than one area.

IV. The Significance of Multiple Representations

The evidence suggests that visual association cortex consists of approximately ten or more separate visual areas. Although there may be subdivisions of visual cortex that do not represent the visual field, all of the areas that have been explored in detail do form systematic representations. Each representation is multiply interconnected with other visual areas. The questions this organization raises are concerned with the phylogeny, the development, and the functions of such a system.

A. Evolution

It is not clear how the multiple representations of the visual field evolved, but a common mechanism of evolution is the duplication of already existing body parts or structures as the result of genetic mutation. After such mutations, the replicated organs can diverge over the course of time in structure and function, and new functions can emerge. It seems possible that the evolution of at least some of the cortical representations may have been by the sudden duplication of already existing visual areas (see Allman and Kaas, 1971a). Another possibility is that mutations caused existing areas to become aberrantly organized, with the duplication of part of the representation and omission of another part. For example, an owl monkey was discovered with a double representation of the upper visual quadrant in DM (Allman and Kaas, 1975). Over generations such a misorganized area presumably could gradually evolve into two complete representations, and thereby create new representations. These two possibilities are alternatives to the more general view that sensory representations gradually differentiated from "unorganized" cortex, or that already organized areas gradually differentiated into additional new areas.

B. Development

The ontogeny of the representations of the retina in visual cortex has not yet been determined. However, the arrangement of aberrantly organized visual areas in Siamese cats (Kaas and Guillery, 1973; Guillery and Kaas, 1971) and an abnormal owl monkey (Allman and Kaas, 1975) suggests that the zero horizontal and vertical meridians are important reference lines in the embryonic development of visual representations. Abnormal reversals of organization within areas occur from the horizontal or the vertical meridian, and it is possible that the organization of each visual area is specified in terms of distance from the horizontal and vertical meridians as well as direction from these reference lines (see Allman and Kaas, 1975).

The matching of visual areas along borders also suggests the importance of the horizontal and vertical meridians as organizing features of visual cortex. Most of the borders of visual areas are formed by the horizontal or the vertical meridians, and adjoining areas match borders. For example, areas like V I and MT with the vertical meridian as most of the outer border are each bounded by a visual area with the inner border formed by the vertical meridian, i.e., V II and DL respectively. On the other hand, the outer borders of other areas such as V II and DL are formed by the horizontal meridian, and along the outer borders along each of these areas there are other visual areas with the representation of the horizontal meridian adjacent to V II or DL. In addition, the common borders of other visual areas are almost completely matching, horizontal meridian to horizontal meridian or vertical meridian to vertical meridian, and the general principle seems to be that representations always match borders in terms of the horizontal or the vertical meridians. To a large extent, bordering areas also match in terms of the portion of the visual field represented along these meridians. Thus, the portion of V I representing 10° in the lower quadrant is bordered by the portion of V II representing 10° in the lower quadrant, and so on. Such matching of parts of the visual field along the horizontal meridian does not always occur, however. Whenever several visual areas border a single area, some mismatch of parts of the field in adjoining areas seems inevitable. DM, for example, forms part of the border of V II, with the horizontal meridian separating the two areas. This particular segment of V II represents only part of the lower visual quadrant, while the adjoining segment of DM represents both the lower and the upper quadrants. Thus, part of DM is mismatched along V II, so that the upper quadrant in DM borders the lower quadrant in V II (see Fig. 4). Borders matched for location in the visual fields have been termed *congruent,* and mismatched borders, *incongruent* (Allman and Kaas, 1975). The large portion of congruent borders suggests that border zones are critical references in the formation of visual representations.

C. Functions

The subdivisions of visual association cortex can be likened to the replicated appendages of the lobster, where structures once very similar in form and function have evolved into structures quite diverse in form and function. The basic premise is that redundancy is not the major role of the multiple visual areas, but rather, the areas are differentially specialized for distinct types of neural processing. Direct evidence of specialization is limited, since the properties of neurons is most of the subdivision of visual cortex have not been studied in any detail. However, Hubel and Wiesel (1970) have presented evidence that many of the neurons in V II are very sensitive to variations in position disparity in an input falling on similar retinal regions of the two eyes, and, presumably, V II is important in stereopsis. In addition, neurons in DM are best activated by stimuli moving at certain rates (Allman and Kaas, 1975), and Zeki (1973) has reported a region of temporal cortex in the rhesus monkey where color-coded cells predominate. Further studies, no doubt, will reveal other examples of specialization.

Given the early model of the visual system as a linear series of connected stations, i.e., retina, lateral geniculate nucleus, V I, V II, V III, and temporal cortex, it was possible to conceive of the visual system as processing input in a strictly serial fashion. Neurons in each station would process incoming information, and then send it on for higher-order processing at the next station. Instead, the multiple areas of visual association cortex and the complexity of the interconnections suggest that neurons in any structure are influenced by many inputs, and the processing may be better characterized as *manifold* rather than serial, although serial, parallel, and hierarchical components of the processing certainly exist.

V. References

Allman, J. M., and Kaas, J. H. 1971a. A representation of the visual field in the caudal third of the middle temporal gyrus of the owl monkey (*Aotus trivirgatus*). *Brain Res.* 31:85–105.

Allman, J. M., and Kaas, J. H. 1971b. Representation of the visual field in striate and adjoining cortex of the owl monkey (*Aotus trivirgatus*). *Brain Res.* 35:89–106.

Allman, J. M., and Kaas, J. H. 1974a. The organization of the second visual area (V II) in the owl monkey: A second order transformation of the visual hemifield. *Brain Res.* 76:247–265.

Allman, J. M., and Kaas, J. H. 1974b. A crescent-shaped cortical visual area surrounding the middle temporal area (MT) in the owl monkey (*Aotus trivirgatus*). *Brain Res.* 81:199–213.

Allman, J. M., and Kaas, J. H. 1975. The dorsomedial cortical visual area: A third tier area in the occipital lobe of the owl monkey (*Aotus trivirgatus*). *Brain Res.* 100:473–487.

Allman, J. M., and Kaas, J. H. 1976. Representation of the visual field on the medial wall of occipital–parietal cortex in the owl monkey. *Science* 191:572–575.

Allman, J. M., Kaas, J. H., and Lane, R. H. 1973. The middle temporal visual area (MT) in the bush baby, *Galago senegalensis*. *Brain Res.* 57:197–202.

Brodmann, K. 1909. *Vergleichende Lokalisationslehre der Grosshirnrinde.* V. A. Barth, Leipzig. Pp. 1–324.

Campbell, A. W. 1905. *Histological Studies on the Localization of Cerebral Function.* Cambridge University Press, Cambridge. 360 pp.

Campos-Ortega, J. A., and Hayhow, W. R. 1972. On the organization of the visual cortical projection to the pulvinar in *Macaca mulatta*. *Brain Behav. Evol.* 6:394–423.

Casagrande, V. A., and Harting, J. K. 1976. Transneuronal transport of ^{3}H fucose and proline in the visual pathways of tree shrew, *Tupaia glis*. *Brain Res.* 96:367–372.

Clark, W. E. Le Gros 1931. The brain of *Microcebus murinus*. *Proc. Zool. Soc. London* 101:463–485.

Clark, W. E. Le Gros 1959. *The Antecedents of Man. An Introduction to the Evolution of the Primates.* Edinburgh University Press, Edinburgh. 374 pp.

Cowey, A. 1964. Projection of the retina onto striate and prestriate cortex in the squirrel monkey, *Saimiri sciureus*. *J. Neurophysiol.* 27:366–396.

Cragg, B. G. 1969. The topography of the afferent projections in the circumstriate visual cortex of the monkey studied by the Nauta method. *Vision Res. 9:*733–747.

Daniel, P. M., and Whitteridge, D. 1961. The representation of the visual field on the cerebral cortex in monkeys. *J. Physiol. (London) 159:*203–221.

Glickstein, M., and Whitteridge, D. 1976. Degeneration of layer III pyramidal cells in area 18 following destruction of callosal input. *Brain Res. 104:*148–151.

Gross, C. G. 1973. Visual functions of inferotemporal cortex. *In* R. Jung (ed.). *Handbook of Sensory Physiology.* Springer, Berlin. Pp. 451–482.

Guillery, R. W., and Kaas, J. H. 1971. A study of normal and congenitally abnormal retinogeniculate terminations in cats. *J. Comp. Neurol. 143:*71–100.

Holländer, H. 1974. Projections from the striate cortex to the diencephalon in the squirrel monkey (*Saimiri sciureus*). A light microscopic radioautographic study following intracortical injection of H^3 leucine. *J. Comp. Neurol. 155:*425–440.

Holmes, G. 1962. Disturbances of vision by cerebral lesions. *J. Physiol. (London) 160:*106–154.

Hubel, D. H. 1975. An autoradiographic study of the retino-cortical projections in the tree shrew (*Tupaia glis*) *Brain Res. 96:*41–50.

Hubel, D. H., and Wiesel, T. N. 1970. Cells sensitive to binocular depth in area 18 of the macaque monkey cortex. *Nature (London) 225:*41–42.

Hubel, D. H., and Wiesel, T. N. 1972. Laminar and columnar distribution of geniculo-cortical fibers in the macaque monkey. *J. Comp. Neurol. 146:*421–450.

Hyvärinen, J., and Poranen, A. 1974. Function of the parietal associative area 7 as revealed from cellular discharges in alert monkeys. *Brain 97:*673–692.

Jones, E. G., and Powell, T. P. S. 1970. An anatomical study of converging sensory pathways within the cerebral cortex of the monkey. *Brain 93:*793–820.

Kaas, J. H., and Guillery, R. W. 1973. The transfer of abnormal visual field representation from the dorsal lateral geniculate nucleus to the visual cortex in Siamese cats. *Brain Res. 59:*61–95.

Kaas, J. H., and Lin, C. S. 1977. Cortical projections of area 18 in owl monkeys. *Vision Res. 16:*739–741.

Kaas, J. H., Lin, C. S., and Casagrande, V. A. 1976. The relay of ipsilation and contralateral retinal input from the lateral geniculate nucleus to striate cortex in the owl monkey. A transneuronal study. *Brain Res. 106:*371–378.

Kaas, J. H., Lin, C. S., and Wagor, E. 1977. Cortical projections of posterior parietal cortex in owl monkeys. *J. Comp. Neurol. 171:*387–408.

Klüver, H., and Bucy, P. C. 1939. Preliminary analysis of functions of the temporal lobes in monkeys. *Arch. Neurol. Psychiat. 42:*979–1000.

Kuypers, H. G. J. M., Szwarcbart, M. K., Mishkin, M., and Rosvold, H. E. 1965. Occipitotemporal corticocortical connections in the rhesus monkey. *Exp. Neurol. 11:*245–262.

Lashley, K. S., and Clark, G. 1946. The cytoarchitecture of the cerebral cortex of *Ateles:* A critical examination of architectonic studies. *J. Comp. Neurol. 85:*223–247.

Le Gros Clark, see Clark.

LeVay, S., Hubel, D. H., and Wiesel, T. N. 1975. The pattern of ocular dominance columns in macaque visual cortex revealed by a reduced silver stain. *J. Comp. Neurol. 159:*559–576.

Lin, C. S., and Kaas, J. H. 1975. Some efferent and afferent connections of a medial division of the inferior pulvinar nucleus in the owl monkey (*Aotus trivirgatus*). *Neurosci. Abstr. 1:*44.

Lin, C. S., and Kaas, J. H. 1977. Projections from cortical visual areas 17, 18, and MT onto the dorsal lateral geniculate nucleus in owl monkeys. *J. Comp. Neurol. 173:*457–474.

Lund, J. S., and Booth, R. G. 1975. Interlaminar connections and pyramidal neuron organization in the visual cortex, area 17, of the macaque monkey. *J. Comp. Neurol. 159:*305–334.

Lund, J. S., Lund, R. D., Hendrickson, A. E., Bunt, A. H., and Fuchs, A. F. 1975. The origin of efferent pathways from the primary visual cortex, area 17, of the macaque monkey as shown by retrograde transport of horseradish peroxidase. *J. Comp. Neurol. 164:*287–303.

Martinez-Millán, M., and Holländer, H. 1975. Cortico-cortical projections for striate cortex of the squirrel monkey (*Saimiri sciureus*). A radioautographic study. *Brain Res. 83:*405–417.

Mishkin, M. 1972. Cortical visual areas and their interactions. *In* A. G. Karczmar and J. C. Eccles (eds.). *The Brain and Human Behavior.* Springer, Berlin. Pp. 187–208.

Mountcastle, V. B. 1975. The view from within: Pathways to the study of perception. *Johns Hopkins Med. J. 136:*109–131.

Myers, R. E. 1965. Commissural connections between occipital lobes of the monkey. *J. Comp. Neurol. 718:*1–16.

Norden, J. J., Lin, C. S., and Kaas, J. H. 1978. Subcortical projections of the dorso-medial visual area (DM) of visual association cortex in the owl monkey, *Aotus trivirgatus. Exp. Brain Res. 32:*1–14.

Polyak, S. 1957. *The Vertebrate Visual System.* University of Chicago Press, Chicago. 1390 pp.

Shoumura, K., Tasashi, A., and Kazuo, K. 1975. Structural organization of "Callosal" OBg in human corpus callosum agenesis. *Brain Res. 93:*241–252.

Smith, G. Elliot. 1907. New studies on the folding of the visual cortex and the significance of the occipital sulci in the human brain. *J. Anat. (London) 41:*198–207.

Solnitzky, O., and Harman, P. J. 1946. The regio occipitalis of the lorisiform lemuroid *Galago demidovii. J. Comp. Neurol. 84:*339–384.

Spatz, W. B. 1975. An efferent connection of the solitary cells of Meynert. A study with horseradish peroxidase in the marmoset, *Callithrix. Brain Res. 92:*450–455.

Spatz, W. B. 1977. Topographically organized reciprocal connections between areas 17 and MT (visual area of superior temporal sulcus) in marmoset *Callithrix jacchus Exp. Brain Res. 27:*559–572.

Spatz, W. B., and Erdmann, G. 1974. Striate cortex projections to the lateral geniculate and other thalamic nuclei; a study using degeneration and autoradiographic tracing methods in the marmoset, *Callithrix. Brain Res. 82:*91–108.

Spatz, W. B., and Tigges, J. 1972. Experimental–anatomical studies on the "Middle

Temporal Visual Area (MT)" in primates. I. Efferent corticocortical connections in the marmoset (*Callithrix jacchus*). *J. Comp. Neurol.* 146:451–464.

Spatz, W. B., and Tigges, J. 1973. Studies on the visual area MT in primates. II. Projection fibers to subcortical structures. *Brain Res.* 61:374–387.

Spatz, W. B., Tigges, J., and Tigges, M. 1970. Subcortical projections, cortical associations and some intrinsic interlaminar connections of the striate cortex in the squirrel monkey (*Saimiri*). *J. Comp. Neurol.* 140:155–174.

Talbot, S. A. 1941. A lateral localization in cat's visual cortex, *Fed. Proc.* 1:84.

Talbot, S. A., and Marshall, W. H. 1941. Physiological studies on neural mechanisms of visual localization and discrimination. *Am. J. Ophthalmol.* 24:1255–1263.

Tigges, J., Spatz, W. B., and Tigges, M. 1973a. Reciprocal point-to-point connections between parastriate and striate cortex in the squirrel monkey (*Saimiri*). *J. Comp. Neurol.* 148:481–490.

Tigges, J., Tigges, M., and Kalaha, C. 1973b. Efferent connections of area 17 in Galago. *Am. J. Phys. Anthropol.* 38:393–398.

Tigges, J., Spatz, W. B., and Tigges M. 1974. Efferent cortico-cortical fiber connections of area 18 in the squirrel monkey (*Saimiri*). *J. Comp. Neurol.* 158:219–236.

Vogt, C., and Vogt, O. 1919. Allgemeine Ergebnisse unserer Hirnforschung. *J. Psychol. Neurol.* 25:279–462.

Wagor, E., Lin, C. S., and Kaas, J. H. 1975. Some cortical projections of the dorsomedial visual area (DM) of association cortex in the owl monkey (*Aotus trivirgatus*). *J. Comp. Neurol.* 163:227–250.

Whitteridge, D. 1973. Projection of optic pathways to visual cortex. *In* R. Jung (ed.). *Handbook of Sensory Physiology*, Vol. VII/3, *Central Processing of Visual Information, Part B. Visual Centers in the Brain.* Springer, Berlin. Pp. 247–268.

Wiesel, T. N., Hubel, D. H., and Lam, D. M. K. 1974. Autoradiographic demonstration of ocular-dominance columns in the monkey striate cortex by means of transneuronal transport. *Brain Res.* 79:273–279.

Wong-Riley, M. T. T. 1974. Demonstration of geniculocortical and callosal projection neurons in the squirrel monkey by means of retrograde axonal transport of horseradish peroxidase. *Brain Res.* 79:267–272.

Woolsey, C. N., and Fairman, D. 1946. Contralateral, ipsilateral and bilateral representation of cutaneous receptors in somatic areas I and II of the cerebral cortex of pig, sheep, and other mammals. *Surgery* 19:684–702.

Zeki, S. M. 1969. Representation of central visual field in prestriate cortex of monkey. *Brain Res.* 14:271–291.

Zeki, S. M. 1970. Interhemispheric connections of prestriate cortex in monkey. *Brain Res.* 19:63–75.

Zeki, S. M. 1971. Cortical projections from two prestriate areas in the monkey. *Brain Res.* 34:19–35.

Zeki, S. M. 1973. Color coding in rhesus monkey prestriate cortex. *Brain Res.* 53:422–427.

Zeki, S. M. 1974. The mosaic organization of the visual cortex in the monkey. *In* R. Bellairs and E. G. Gray (eds.). *Essays on the Nervous System—A Festschrift for Professor J. Z. Young.* Clarendon Press, Oxford. Pp. 327–343.

8

The Relevance of Endocasts for Studying Primate Brain Evolution

Ralph L. Holloway

I. Introduction

The most proximal evidence for brain evolution within any taxonomic group of animals is from paleoneurology, the study of brain endocasts. The higher primates, however, i.e., pongids and hominids, have a notorious reputation for not being too faithful in leaving solid, interpretable evidence on the surface of their endocasts. Whether this is because they are relatively large-brained creatures or simply phyletically perverse and spiteful in character, preferring that their brain phylogeny remain unknown because of meningeal tissues' conspiring to eradicate all decent gyral and sulcal configurations, is unknown at present. Certainly the first factor, large brain size, is in all likelihood paramount. In any event, except for a *very few* exceptional cases in both chimpanzees and humans, the cortical gyri and sulci are covered by thick meninges and

RALPH L. HOLLOWAY • Department of Anthropology, Columbia University, New York, New York 10027.

usually do not imprint their forms on the internal table of bone of the cranium.*

To become a bit more serious, however, I would like to review briefly the status of endocasts in understanding hominid brain evolution, if not modern pongid evolution, and suggest, on the basis of current research, some directions for the future.

II. Possible Lines of Evidence for Brain Evolution

Two particular aspects of neuroanatomy have tremendous relevance to both general and specific questions as to how animal brains evolve(d): (1) neural mass, and (2) how neural masses are "wired." Other relevant aspects are the remaining peripheral functional anatomy of the animals and the kinds of environments in which they interact with their growing and "behaving" brains. That is, if we are wont to talk about "language" and Broca's area, or the inferior parietal lobule, we must keep in mind any and all evidence regarding laryngeal and pharyngeal relationships—tongue, palate, sinuses, etc.—and the spectrum of social behavioral repertoires that characterize the species under study. Nor can we talk about mass and wiring in any holistic sense without reflecting upon and taking into consideration how brains become programmed to interact and adapt within differing social and material environments. Endocasts may indeed be the most proximal source of direct evidence for brain evolution, but in higher primates the "proximalness" relates almost completely to mass,† and not "wiring." Only comparative neuroanatomy, necessarily limited to the current end products of various lines of evolution, can provide direct evidence about

* It is a piteous sight to see the expressions on the faces of students when, after having named all the gyri and sulci on primate brain photographs or real specimens, they are confronted with endocasts of apes and humans and asked to find the lunate and central sulci, the supramarginal gyrus, etc., etc. I can only point out to them that their despair has been shared by some very great personages in the neurosciences (e.g., Smith, Keith, Le Gros Clark, von Bonin). Indeed, I have discovered that after ten years of endocast study some levity is essential to good health; hence this Introduction.

† At least for the present. It is hoped that the future holds more promise, already suggested by the research of LeMay (1976) on cerebral asymmetries in pongids, Dewson's (1976) work on auditory asymmetry in monkeys, and LeMay and Geschwind's (1977) finding of temporal lobe asymmetry in chimpanzees. See also Yeni-Komshian and Benson (1976) for evidence of left–right asymmetry of the Sylvian fissure.

how different brains are wired. We study the extant animals' brains to understand how neural variation in the organization of neural mass and fiber tracts (wiring) contribute to behavioral variation, and from these studies general and specific principles are derived which we apply to whatever lines of evolutionary development we are considering. Thus it is possible, for example, to combine knowledge from neurophysiological mappings of sensory and motor responses with endocasts from several lines of mammalian evolution, as Radinsky has so beautifully demonstrated (Radinsky, 1968, 1970, 1971, 1974a,b, 1975a,b), putting to rest once and for all the old shibboleth that endocasts are useless for understanding brain evolution. Radinsky's work on *Aegyptopithecus* shows that there is indeed some usefulness to Tertiary (Oligocene) primitive pongid endocasts (Radinsky, 1974b), and that of his students (e.g., Falk, 1976) on cercopithecoid brains also shows promise of demonstrating sulcal and gyral changes within certain taxa of these primates.

In Radinsky's (1974b) work on pongid endocasts, both *Aegyptopithecus* (Oligocene) and *Dryopithecus africanus* (Miocene—formerly known as "Proconsul africanus") were clearly small-brained creatures, and, despite the fragmentary nature of the cranial remains, some level of gyral and sulcal relief remained unhidden, a circumstance very rare in the extant larger-brained pongids and hominids. Whether size of brain alone is sufficient to account for gyral and sulcal replication is doubtful. All of the *Homo erectus* endocasts from Indonesia and China tend to show relief on the frontal lobe but not elsewhere (Shellshear and Smith, 1934). The Taung endocast, of what was supposedly a gracile *Australopithecus*, shows considerable relief (Schepers, 1946, 1950, 1952; Le Gros Clark, 1947; Dart, 1956; Holloway, 1974, 1975a) on frontal, parietal, temporal, and occipital lobes, which is not uncommon for young animals within the Hominoidea. Even SK1585 (Holloway, 1972b), a robust australopithecine, shows some gyral and sulcal relief, albeit far less than the Taung specimen. O.H.5, from Olduvai, shows none (Tobias, 1971). All of the East African specimens, however, (see Holloway, 1972a,b, 1973a,b, 1975a,b,) including both Olduvai Gorge and Lake Turkana (formerly Lake Rudolf), have been eroded so that little if any gyral and sulcal patterns can be safely identified. These latter specimens include early *Homo, Homo erectus* (e.g., ER 3733, O.H. 9), and both gracile and robust *Australopithecus*. Neanderthal specimens show some evidence for fissuration in the frontal lobe, but none elsewhere. In short, relief patterns are probably multifactorially determined, involving a complex mix of brain size, age, and taxonomic grouping.

What, then, can be learned from such a plurality of groups and variability of convolutional impressions?

There are at least five "levels" of useful evidence to be gleaned from endocasts, depending both on their completeness and replicability of cortical details. I make no claims that the following schema is complete or without some arbitrariness. It will, I hope, serve to illustrate certain points, strengths, and weaknesses about what can be expected from hominoid endocasts. The limitations will be discussed more fully later.

Level 1 is simply gross brain size, i.e., the volume of neural mass (with attending dural tissues, ventricles, cerebrospinal fluid, etc.) confined by the internal table of bone of the cranium. This parameter, or "statistic" as Jerison (1973) prefers to call it, has a number of obvious uses. (1) It is the most direct measurement of the organism's brain size and can be reasonably translated into units of weight since the specific gravity of neural tissue is essentially 1.0. (2) It is indispensable for calculating subsidiary statistics, *such as relative brain size* (brain size/brain weight) and degree or amount of *encephalization,* i.e., the E.Q. (or encephalization quotient) between the actual brain size and that theoretically expected for an animal of a certain body weight, usually based on a previously defined allometric relation (or regression) between log brain weight and log body weight, based on some particular group of animal taxa. Naturally, body weights, or some careful approximation to them, are necessary for these two latter statistics. (3) Brain volume or weight probably has intrinsic relationships to other kinds of neural and basic biological variables, such as neuron size, neural density, possibly glial/neural ratios, dendritic branching, schedules of neurological events such as hyperplasia, hypertrophy, and myelination, life span, metabolic rates, behavioral variables, and, of course, time itself. The last, time, becomes of very great theoretical interest since with a reasonably full fossil record the trends, either continuous or discontinuous, with spurts or lags, all provide essential clues to selection pressures in the past for neural mass (for example, see Holloway, 1972a for diagrams) and provide data for calculating evolutionary rates. (For reviews of some of the possibilities of relationships between brain size and other biological variables, see Jerison, 1973; Sacher, 1970;

Holloway, 1968.) (4) As with any other morphological unit, brain endocasts can be studied morphometrically. That is, the size–shape relationships within and between taxa can be analyzed using a variety of uni- and multivariate statistical procedures, some of which will be described further on. These analyses can be done on problems of regional variation (e.g., different lobes) and asymmetries, i.e., left, right.

Level 2 might be termed areal determination, that is, how the surface of the endocast was divided up into major lobar regions, such as the frontal, parietal, temporal, occipital, and cerebellar. This level of analysis, of course, depends on accurate delineation of those sulcal patterns which neuroanatomists use to define lobe boundaries: the central or rolandic sulcus, the rhinal sulcus, the Sylvian sulcus, and the lunate sulcus or "affenspalte," all of which, the Sylvian excepted, offer great difficulties in extant hominoid endocasts. At the risk of a Panglossian view, such identification would allow for accurate demonstration of major lobe areas, which could be related to brain size in some mathematical way. The number of literature citations possible in which the frontal lobe is viewed as having increased in size, relatively, during hominoid evolution is very great, and interestingly not a single whit of unambiguous quantification is demonstrable. (See Holloway, 1968, for a review of this research.) Even Radinsky (1974b, 1975c) claims that Dryopithecus and Aegyptopithecus have relatively smaller frontal lobes than extant pongids on fragmentary endocasts. This is a question of both allometry and the reliability of gestalt impressions. That is, almost all observations on this question are purely qualitative. The neuroanatomical evidence does not suggest relative increase in frontal lobe, although it does for the parietal and posterior aspects of the temporal lobe and a relative diminution in visual striate cortex on the lateral surface.

Another aspect of this level which has more recently received some well-needed attention is the question of local asymmetries, e.g., differences in the length of the Sylvian fissure between right and left sides, width of occipital poles, ventricular size, occipital and frontal petalias, etc. (LeMay, 1976, 1977). This work is being done both on radiographs of extant human and pongid brains and examination of fossil endocasts. (For a review of past studies and most recent investigations, see particularly LeMay, 1976, 1977.) While many asymmetries have been noted, particularly for extant brains, two problems present themselves in terms of the fossil record. First, the functional significance of the asymmetries is not fully known, and, second unambiguous and quantitatively demonstrable asymmetries on the fossil hominoid endocasts are very difficult given the often incomplete nature of the material. Nevertheless, as our understanding of the functional picture becomes clearer, i.e., the relationship of these gross asymmetries to handedness, cerebral dominance, and sensory, motor, and language functioning, this level of analysis may hold considerably more promise for evolutionary studies on the brain than realized before.

Level 3 is related to major sulcal and gyral identifications and meningeal blood vessel patterns which appear to show some taxonomic constancy (Saban, 1976, 1977). The former are of course related to level 2 but can also be studied in their own right with regard to their variations and changes with time, aiding with broad taxonomic distinctions and helping to delineate and lend interpretation to neurophysiological interpretation of sensorimotor functioning.

Level 4 relates to the identification of secondary and tertiary sulcal and gyral convolutions making up the external cortical morphology of body functional regions, such as the third inferior frontal convolution (Broca's area), Wernices' area, dorsal frontal eye movement fields, primary visual striate cortex, lateral extensions of the calcarine fissure, superior temporal gyrus, auditory area, etc. A beautiful example of this level of analysis is Welker and Campos's (1963) and Radinsky's (1968, 1975a,b) work on the evolution of the procyonids and pinniped carnivores, which relates to:

Level 5 where secondary and tertiary convolutions can be related to explicitly functional paradigms based on neurophysiological mappings of the cerebral cortex of different animals.

Level 6 does not really exist but would, if logically pursued, relate to subcortical relationships, *inferred* from our knowledge of comparative neuroanatomy and corticosubcortical interrelationships. For example, if one could quantitatively demonstrate both a relative and absolute increase in the amount of inferior parietal cortical tissue among a group of fossil endocasts evolutionarily related, one could infer that the pulvinar nucleus of the thalamus underwent some concomitant increase in mass, with attending elaboration of corticothalamic and corticocortical interconnections.

Each of these levels of observation and description carries its own level of functional interpretation as well, and the goal of any study based on endocasts is to provide as holistic an interpretation as possible, based both on comparative studies of extant animals and the remaining fossil evidence aside from endocasts. In broad strokes, our understanding of the evolutionary changes that led to the emergence of *Homo*, perhaps between two and three million years ago, rests on a reticulation of the evolution of locomotion (upright bipedal striding gait), utilization of the hands for manipulating the environment (social and material) as partially evidenced by the appearance in the fossil record of stone tools made to standardized patterns, the elaboration of communicative skills, most probably involving both verbal and nonverbal modalities, hand–eye coordination, associative reasoning skills, etc. To the extent that these broad levels of form–environmental adaptation are understood, the endocasts of hominoids are studied within these frameworks, and as much qualitative and quantitative information as can be gleaned from examination of levels 1–5 from the endocast surfaces is related to our *a priori* assumptions regarding past evolutionary trends.

III. Qualitative and Quantitative Descriptions

Most of the research done in primate (and other animal) paleoneurology is necessarily of a qualitative nature which can, and often does, incorporate each of the first five levels of description mentioned above—that is, whether gyrus *x* or sulcus *y* can be seen, whether the frontal lobe is relatively small or large (or small*er* or larg*er* than *z*), whether the primary visual striate cortex is expanded or not, or whether or not the olfactory bulbs are reduced. Statements are couched in terms of absence or presence, smaller or larger. Occasionally, the quantitative description will include level 1, brain endocast size, if the specimen is complete enough, and might include topographical mensuration of the nature of map coordinates, e.g., ". . . the coronal sulcus is 3 mm long, situated approximately 13 mm from the caudal end of the endocast. . . ." These kinds of statements are indispensable descriptions but, aside from level 1, do not of themselves provide data for morphometric analysis and *unambiguous* phylogenetic interpretation, except in the sense of taxonomic identification. Even these minimal descriptions run afoul of at least four facts of paleontological life: (1) specimens are seldom complete, unbroken, or undistorted; (2) the internal table of cranial bone often is exfoliative; (3) larger-brained specimens do not give fine details of gyral and sulcal relief; and (4) sample sizes are ridiculously low so there seldom, if ever, exist any good indications of variability.

A fifth stumbling block is that the scientist doing the description is particularly skilled and his colleagues are not, or there are so few scientists working with endocasts that most descriptive statements are taken on faith. Two examples might suffice to make this point, one from my own work on *Australopithecus* and one from Radinsky's (1974b) study of the Oligocene *Aegyptopithecus*. (Remember, I am talking about unambiguous demonstration of levels, not whether the various statements made are actually true or false.) In some recent publications (1974, 1975a, 1976) I tried to argue that at least some of the hominid australopithecine endocasts showed a morphological pattern demonstrably hominid and not pongid, aside from any considerations of gross size of the endocast. Levels 2–5 were used, wherein claims of the following sort were made: In Taung and SK 1585 (supposedly a gracile and a robust australopithecine respectively) the lunate sulcus was oriented posteriorly; there appeared to be more fissuration in total than in pongid endocasts; the anterior tips of the temporal lobes were of human shape; the cerebellar lobes looked more hominid than pongid. I believe these statements to be true, but they have not been *unambiguously* demonstrated and are thus open to doubt and independent study. Radinsky (1974b, 1975c) has claimed that in *Aegyptopithecus* the central or coronal sulcus is identifiable and that the frontal lobe appears to be smaller, relatively, than in extant pongids. I believe Radinsky is correct about the central sulcus, although I personally have difficulty seeing it on the endocast and feeling convinced it is indeed the central, not the precentral or an artifact of the fractured and incomplete nature of the cranial remains.

As to the relative size of the frontal lobe, this is hardly *unambiguously* demonstrable, given that (1) we must accept the central sulcus where Radinsky claims it is if we are to measure the frontal lobe, and (2) one cannot get a completely accurate volume of the whole endocast or the frontal because of incompleteness. In fact, those of us who study paleoneurology are more often than not reduced to leaving the argument in the form of "... if not x, then where (else) or what (else) is x?" This is not the most enviable position to be in, scientifically, yet the phylogenetic interpretations we all wish for must necessarily depend heavily on these levels of analysis.

In the next section I would like to discuss some possible examples of how greater information might be secured from endocasts, using some current examples from my own research on hominid brain endocast evolution.

IV. Toward Fuller Morphometric Analyses

In the last ten years, I have been pursuing two goals in the study of hominoid endocasts: (1) to use morphometric data from a large sample of different pongid and hominid endocasts to enable unambiguous demonstration of taxonomic affinity, *independent of brain size* (i.e., on the basis of shape); (2) to relate differences in morphometry between various taxa to functional and evolutionary relationships. The basic question is: are there species-specific morphometric patterns that can be gleaned from a sufficient body of mensurational data on endocasts to allow analysis of goals (1) and (2)? As almost all mensurational data have some strong allometric relationship to gross endocast size, the questions I am currently trying to test are whether or not the *residuals* from allometric relationships show species-specific patterns that are informationally useful for both taxonomic identification and functional interpretation.

Two studies are currently in progress, and as they are not yet completed the descriptions that follow should only be considered tentative and preliminary, and I mention these studies *only* to give some idea and examples of newer directions being taken in endocast studies.

A. Study 1

In this study, based on a sample of 40 *Pan paniscus*, 33 *Pan troglodytes*, 39 *Gorillas*, 6 *Homo sapiens*, and all the available fossil hominid endocasts, but *not* including so-called Neanderthals, 19 basic measurements were taken, including volume. These measurements are nothing more than crude linear arc and chord distances between various points on the endocast surface, which provide information about size and shape. The following are examples of such measurements: chord lengths between frontal and occipital poles, and both lateral and dorsal arc lengths between these same points; greatest width (usually on superior temporal gyrus) of the endocast, measuring both arc and chord distances; height of endocast from vertex to lowest temporal lobe projection; height, width, and length of cerebellar lobes. Included are a number of measurements between anthropometric landmarks, such as basion–bregma, bregma–lambda, biasterionic breadth, bregma–asterion, again both in chord and arc form. From these basic 19 measurements, of which the above are only a sample, some 37 indices have been constructed to provide ratios of arc-to-chord measures, suited, we hope, to measure curvature as well as the more traditional ratios, e.g., length to breadth and height to length.

It should be apparent that these measurements are not functionally designed but are merely ways of characterizing the space confined by the outer boundary of the endocast. Consequently, one should only expect size and shape characteristics of the various taxa to result from any statistical analyses of these data and not functional, neurobiological, evolutionary statements. What are being measured, literally, are the inside dimensions of the cranium and not functionally definable entities. To the extent that the crania themselves differ in shape taxonomically, these measurements and indices help define those shape and size changes with greater precision than most gestalt descriptions.

I have purposely italicized the above comments for the reader's benefit and to underline the limitations of this very traditional way of measuring the endocasts. Scattered throughout the literature, one can find references to various endocast indices that purportedly demonstrate level 2 relationships, i.e., major lobe size changes (see for example von Bonin, 1963; Schepers, 1950, 1952; and Holloway, 1964, 1968, for a review of these indices). These are almost always based on lateral projections to a two-dimensional surface, and decisions as to the exact location of most of the major sulci (Sylvian and central) are made on the basis of educated guesses rather than actual demonstration. This is an important limitation. These data, however, are not projections but actual measurements and provide the advantage of being suitable for a number of essential and interesting statistical manipulations. In addition, the comparative base, the pongids, are over 90 in number, giving valuable information on the ranges and nature of size and shape variations.

I will not go into the details of statistical analyses here, as their data are still in a preliminary stage, but the following will show some of the directions taken and their significance and limitations.

Needless to say, if one is interested in size–shape differences and interactions, one must first see to what extent the measurements and indices are allometrically related to the volume of the endocast. It is not surprising, of course, that each of the basic 19 measurements is highly correlated to volume, the correlation, r, being anywhere from .85 to .98, when plotted in log–log terms. Similarly, a number of the indices are likewise related to volume with various degrees of correlation and significance. By correcting for allometry, one can then test, particularly through Anova and discriminant analysis, whether the *residuals*, the differences between the expected allometric and actual values, have any taxonomic information. Or, one can use factor analysis to take out size as the first principal component, and try discriminant analysis on the remaining factor scores.

What appears to be the case is that, indeed, there is taxonomic information available in the residuals, and depending on the variables chosen—whether the discriminant analyses are forced or stepwise, whether prior probabilities of taxon membership are equal, adjusted by size, or theoretical probabilities are used (e.g., one would not expect the KNM-ER 1470 2.6-million-year-old *Homo* endocast to have *any* probability of being in the pongid groups)—discriminant analysis gives 75–90% correct classifications; the factor scores, of which 14 emerge, all make some sort of geometric, morphometric sense, such as size, dorsal curvature, lateral curvature, the relation between dorsal and lateral curvature, height relative to volume, breadth and height of the cerebellar lobes relative to the cerebral part of the endocast, biasterionic chord–arc ratios, etc. When size is added as a factor, the classifications of course go up to 100%, even with the vast overlapping between the two *Pan* and *Gorilla* taxa, and those of *Australopithecus africanus* and *Australopithecus robustus*.

There is yet one other set of reasons for doing these kinds of morphometric studies. In some instances, endocasts are variably incomplete, and, to whatever degree there exist lawful mathematical relationships between volume and the various measurements, and intercorrelations among the measurements, it is possible to establish *predictor equations* to aid in reconstructing the missing endocast portions or to establish confidence limits for multiple regressions to find the total volume of the endocasts. Some of these results have been described in Holloway (1978) and will not be documented again here.

In sum, thus far this study indicates two promising things: (1) the residuals from allometric corrections have taxonomic value, particularly in multivariate statistical analyses, and thus provide a highly accurate basis for assigning taxonomic designations; (2) the data are useful toward more careful prediction of other measurements. As for the question of functional interpretation, I do not regard these data, as far as they have been analyzed, of any real value until such time as our understanding of the relation of geometrical form to functioning is better developed.

B. Study 2

The problems of the measurements taken in Study 1 are that only those that are replicable (meaning easily defined) can be taken, and they do not have functional definition. What is needed is some system where individual measurements on each gyrus and sulcus can be obtained, compared, and demonstrated unequivocally, which is no small problem.

A number of pilot studies are now underway utilizing a different mensuration technique. Using a polar-coordinate stereoplotter devised by Oyen and Walker (1977), it has been possible to collect 325 data points on the dorsal surface alone of each endocast. To date, we have collected close to 15,000 data points for statistical analysis. The sample for this study is only 45 endocasts, about equally divided among 9 taxa of hominoids, i.e., about five endocasts per taxon (*Pan paniscus, Pan, troglodytes, Pan gorilla, Homo sapiens, Australopithecus africanus, Australopithecus robustus, Homo erectus* from Indonesia and China, and *Homo sapiens soloensis*). Endocasts of KNM-ER 1813, 1805, 1470, and OH 9 (see Holloway, 1975a,b) are used as well but not initially classified.

The procedure consists of placing the endocast in the stereoplotter apparatus with base down, dorsal surface exposed above the equator of the instrument, the plane of the horizontal (or equator) passing exactly through both frontal and occipital poles, and the endocast positioned so that the center is defined as the midway point between frontal and occipital poles. (These points were chosen as standardized landmarks because we surely regard them as anatomically and functionally homologous.) Attached to the horizontal plate of the apparatus (which freely revolves through 360° is a vertical arc with a pointer freely slidable along the horizontal and vertical arc through 180°. Thus, by varying both the horizontal and vertical components, *a radial distance from the center of the endocast to the surface can be taken.* These radial distances thus have two angular coordinates. Depending on one's tolerance, patience, and compulsiveness, one can take measurements from any point on the dorsal surface desired, or one can take measurements every so many degrees. To date, we have been collecting data points every 10° on the dorsal surface.

There are many things that can be done with these data. They can be mapped, giving contour maps of the distances or intervals of change between successive points; "average" (per taxon) maps can be drawn and compared with other taxon maps; the points can be selectively chosen along either vertical or horizontal transects and treated in a number of statistical ways. Finally, actual brains, or casts thereof, can be measured in the same way to form a basis of control for studying the endocasts. *The reason for this, and indeed its strength, is that in polar coordinates allometric relationships insure a higher degree of constancy of location than in other coordinates and thus better (less equivocally) identify these areas on the endocasts.*

I do not pretend at this time in our studies using these techniques that the sample sizes are adequate, that the volume of data points is not a distinct example of mathematical "overkill" that correspondences between all cortical gyri and sulcal patterns on actual brains and endocasts are perfect, or that we will be able to demonstrate level 2–5 changes in evolutionary development with perfection. Still, I believe this technique holds very great promise for coming close to such Panglossian goals and should, minimally, provide quantitative, rather than qualitative, statements about local topographical changes on the endocast surfaces which can be reasonably related to functional knowledge.

To date, some eight pilot studies have been run on the data given by this sample of 45 endocasts, divided into nine groups. Angular transects have been taken every 20°, from anterior to posterior along the vertical orientation, i.e., starting with a point on the horizontal surface 20° from the midsagittal plane and going upward to the vertex of the endocast. This yields 10 points (for each 10°) for each side of the endocast. If we were to choose horizontal transects, the number of points, anterior to posterior, would be 19. Aside from the horizontal and sagittal transects which are both 19 points, we have chosen to do pilot studies on the 10-point vertical transects because the number of variables is approximately equal to the number of taxonomic groups.

The logarithm of each point (radial distance) for each endocast

(N = 45) is regressed against the logarithm of the endocast's volume. The correlation is very high, with r varying between .92 and .98. Each point thus has its own allometric equation, and this equation is then used to derive the *residuals*, which we call DIFFS 1–10 (or DIFFS 1–19 if using horizontal transects). In addition, the intervals between adjacent points are collected to give information of velocity of slope changes. For example, if the radial distance of point 1 is 55 mm and point 2 adjacent is 58 mm, the change is 3 mm per 10° arc through that transect, and so on, each subtraction being done between adjacent points.

Again, we are interested in the two possibilities mentioned previously regarding taxonomic shape patterns and functional interpretation. At this stage of the pilot analyses, however, the endeavor is to test only for shape differences that can be useful for taxonomic classification.

At this point it would be well to point out that one is obliged to test the residuals against the logarithm of volume in order to ensure that these residuals are not themselves allometrically related to volume. This has been done in all instances through the SPSS Anova program, where each DIFF is the dependent variable, the taxonomic group is the independent variable, and log volume is the covariate. There are, out of eight pilot studies, no really significant allometric relationships between the DIFFS and log volume. This fact permits both the Anova and Oneway statistical routines to be used and ensures that when discriminant analysis is used size will not affect classifications.

Again, I will only briefly indicate the major outlines of the results so far. All posterior transects, i.e., posterior 20°, 40°, 60°, show greater classification scores in discriminant analysis, at around 85 to 90%, and the highest loadings (coefficients) are usually those points closest to the horizontal plane. The classification scores for anterior transects are somewhat lower, but not uniformly so. In addition, the F-ratios have their highest significance for taxonomic effects on the same points. These transects really involve the inferior parietal, superior and posterior temporal, and anterior occipital regions of the endocasts. The F-ratios are currently being plotted, transect by transect, to give a mapping of where the highest and lowest values occur over the dorsal endocast surface. In general, the same results occur with both the horizontal and sagittal transects, which have 19 points. Expectedly, the classification scores from discriminant analyses are higher, since the number of variables is about double that of all other angular transects. Incidentally, most misclassifications occur between *Pan paniscus* and

Pan troglodytes, and between the two *Homo erectus* groups from Indonesia and China. Interestingly, the australopithecine groups and Modern *Homo sapiens* tend to classify at 100%. Needless to say, larger sample sizes, for testing both classified and unclassified (but known) endocasts are necessary, and larger samples are currently being examined.

In summary, Study 2 pilot studies suggest, but hardly prove at this early date, that point-by-point analysis of the dorsal endocast surface certainly has taxonomic information that helps to discriminate shape features between both widely and narrowly separated hominid and pongid groups and that these differences are strongest in the posterior regions of the endocasts. It is encouraging from the functional point of view, since it is these regions which most neurobiologists suspect have undergone evolutionary reorganization, involving a relative decrease in lateral extent of primary visual striate cortex and an expansion of parietal and temporal lobe association cortex. The sample sizes for each group, however, are very small, and until these are larger, at least for the modern extant species of pongids and *Homo,* these indications, while promising, must await further validation.

V. Addendum

The making of an endocast is basically a quite simple procedure, and the author is innocent of any methodological invention in this area, as the basic technique was published by Radinsky (1968) and apparently independently reinvented by Murrill and Wallace (1971). Essentially, a cranium is filled with liquid or viscous latex such that all possible anatomical details existing on the internal table of cranial bone are filled or covered with the latex. This is usually achieved by first closing off all cranial foramina temporarily with plasticene or some other malleable substance and rotating the cranium or skull while the latex is inside. After this, the excess nonadhering latex is poured out through the foramen magnum, and the cranium is vigorously shaken to distribute the latex evenly without forming local, thickened, pools. This layer, the first, is allowed to dry thoroughly, usually by forcing a jet of warm or cool air into the foramen magnum with a hairdryer or other suitable equipment. After this layer has dried, the cranium is refilled with latex and the process outlined above is repeated as many times as necessary to achieve a total layer of approximately 1 to 2 mm thickness. The number of repetitions will obviously depend on the original viscosity of the latex and on the size of the specimen. I prefer to use a thinner solution than others (e.g., Radinsky, personal communication; . Falk, 1976), and I generally attempt five or six pourings. A thicker fluid can reduce the pourings to one or two sufficient layers.

After the layers of latex have dried, the whole (cranium with dried latex) is put into an oven at approximately 50° to 70°C for 3 or 4 hours, which further dries the latex and cures it. This operation, incidentally, while perhaps sounding dreadful to museum keepers, does not in any way damage the specimens, whether fossil or recent.

After the specimen has been layered with latex and cured, the problem of extracting the latex shell begins. Simply, this means collapsing the latex shell or mold inside of the cranium and extracting it through some suitably-sized foramen or fissure, usually the foramen magnum. The latex does not "stick" to the cranial wall but separates quite easily from it. Potential problems are that (1) in collapsing, the interior surfaces of latex can stick to each other, and so can the external surface; (2) delicate structures of intracranial anatomy, for example, the anterior and posterior clinoid processes of the sella turcica, the cribriform plate, the foramen lacerum and jugular complex, or certain of the cranial sutures, particularly in young specimens can provide some difficulty or obstacles to the easy extraction of the latex shell.

The first problem, that of self-adhesion, is very simply overcome by applying either water or talc (I use baby powder) into the inside of the latex shell *and* between the latex shell and cranial bone while collapsing the endocast. The second problem is overcome by being very careful to cover properly all foramina *before* pouring the latex and by exercising great care in collapsing the latex shell away from the areas mentioned above. If there is some element of skill or expertise involved in this simple process, it is here.

Once the endocast is collapsed inside the cranium and carefully manipulated out through the foramen magnum, the technician will experience the delightful and happy sensations of seeing, hearing, and feeling the latex shell literally popping back to its original *in situ* form, with all conceivable detail dutifully and faithfully imprinted on the external surface.

This basically describes the technique for complete crania. Fossil and otherwise fragmentary specimens require some modifications in technique depending on their own idiosyncratic conditions and the ultimate purpose of making the endocast in the first place. Normally, dimensional accuracy is highly desired, so that accurate measurements of volume, surface area, or linear distances can be taken. This requires stabilizing the dimensions of the endocast immediately upon extraction from the cranial portion. This can be done in at least two basic ways: (1) by filling the endocast with liquid plaster of Paris while immersed in water and allowing to harden; (2) by filling the latex shell *in situ* in the cranium, with plaster, and taking the cranium apart along the sutures or cracks.

The first method is usually done with complete, extant, recent specimens and those fossil specimens which are complete and strong enough to allow the latex shell to be removed from the foramen magnum or basal opening. The second method works very well with fragmented fossil specimens glued together along their cracked joints. For example, the hominid specimens from Lake Turkana, Kenya, such as KNM-E-R 1470, 1805, 1813, 3733, and 3883, were done in just this way, yielding dimensionally perfect endocasts with absolutely no damage to the original specimens.

It is, I hope, obvious that all of the above descriptions apply only to the basics of the techniques, for it is a fact, as anyone who has made these endocasts has experienced, that each specimen requires some individual attention, special effort and care, and heaps of concentration and variable time. Sometimes it is possible to make several endocasts a day; on the other hand, endocasting the infamous ER 1470 early *Homo* cranium took several days, two or three of which were spent just in planning how to make the endocast without jeopardizing the integrity of the specimen or sacrificing dimensional perfection or anatomical detail.

Measuring the volume of an endocast is similarly a simple process, which can be done either by weighing the volume of water displaced by immersion of the endocast, by weighing the loss of weight of the endocast when immersed (e.g., Jerison, 1973), or only visually by determining volume displacement in a graduated cylinder or beaker. I prefer the first method and use a beaker fitted with a narrow tube and spout through which the excess water can be collected during immersion. Variation of readings by the first two methods is usually within 1 or 2 ml for large-volumed animals (viz., *Homo*), and within 1 ml for smaller forms (e.g., *Pan* or *Gorilla*).

(For further information regarding these techniques, reconstructions, and empirical data on fossil hominids, see Holloway, 1970a,b, 1972a,b, 1973a,b, 1975a,b, 1978.)

VI. References

Clark, W. E. Le Gros, 1947. Observations on the anatomy of the fossil Austral-opithecinae. *J. Anat. 81:*300.

Dart, R. A. 1956. The relationship of brain size and brain pattern to human status. *S. Afr. J. Med. Sci. 21:*23.

Dewson, J. H. 1976. Preliminary evidence of hemispheric asymmetry of auditory functions in monkeys. *In* S. Harnad *et al.* (ed.). *Lateralization in the Nervous System.* Academic Press, New York. Pp. 63–74.

Dimond, S. J., and Beaumont, J. G. (eds.). 1974. *Hemisphere Function in the Human Brain.* Paul Elek, London.

Falk, D. D. 1976. External neuroanatomy of the Cercopithecoidea. Ph.D. Thesis, University of Michigan, Ann Arbor.

Holloway, R. L. 1964. Some aspects of quantitative relations in the primate brain. Unpublished Ph.D. Dissertation. University of California, Berkeley.

Holloway, R. L. 1968. The evolution of the primate brain: Some aspects of quantitative relations. *Brain Res. 7:*121–172.

Holloway, R. L. 1970a. New endocranial values for the australopithecines. *Nature 227:*199–200.

Holloway, R. L. 1970b. Australopithecine endocast (Taung specimen, 1924): A new volume determination. *Science 168:*966–968.

Holloway, R. L. 1972a. Australopithecine endocasts, brain evolution in the Hominoidea and a model of hominid evolution. *In* R. H. Tuttle (ed.). *The Functional and Evolutionary Biology of Primates.* Aldine Press, Chicago. Pp. 185–204.

Holloway, R. L. 1972b. New australopithecine endocast, SK1585, from Swartkrans, S. Africa. *Am. J. Phys. Anthropol. 37:*173–186.

Holloway, R. L. 1973a. New endocranial values for the East African early hominids. *Nature 243:*97–99.

Holloway, R. L. 1973b. Endocranial capacities of the early African hominids and the role of the brain in human mosaic evolution. *J. Hum. Evol.* (Dart Memorial Volume) *2:*449–450.

Holloway, R. L. 1974. The casts of fossil hominid brains. *Sci. Am. 231*(1):6–115.

Holloway, R. L. 1975a. 43rd James Arthur Lecture at the American Museum of Natural History, on the Evolution of the Human Brain, The role of human social behavior in the evolution of the brain, 1973. American Museum of Natural History.

Holloway, R. L. 1975b. Early hominid endocasts: Volumes, morphology, and significance. *In* R. H. Tuttle (ed.). *Primate Functional Morphology and Evolution.* Mouton Press, Hague. Pp. 393–416.

Holloway, R. L. 1976. Paleoneurological evidence for language origins. *In* S. R. Harnad, H. D. Steklis, and J. Lancaster (eds.). Origins and Evolution of Language and Speech. *Ann. N.Y. Acad. Sci. 280:*330–348.

Holloway, R. L. 1978. Some problems of hominid brain endocast reconstruction, allometry, and neural reorganization, to appear in Colloquium VI of the IX Congress of U.I.S.S.P.P., Nice, 1976 Congress. In press.

Jerison, H. 1973. *Evolution of the Brain and Intelligence.* Academic Press, New York.

Le Gros Clark, see Clark.

LeMay, M. 1975. The language capability of Neanderthal man. *Am. J. Phys. Anthropol. 42:*9–14.

LeMay, M. 1976. Morphological cerebral asymmetries of modern man, fossil man, and non-human primate. *In* S. R. Harnad, H. D. Steklis, J. Lancaster (eds.). Origins and Evolution of Language and Speech, *Ann. N.Y. Acad. Sci. 280:*349–360.

LeMay, M. 1977. Asymmetries of the skull and handedness. *J. Neurol. Sci. 32:*243–253.

LeMay, M., and Culebras, A. 1972. Human brain-morphological differences in the hemispheres demonstrable by carotid arteriography. *N. Eng. J. Med. 287:*168–70.

LeMay, M., and Geschwind, N. 1978. Asymmetries of the human cerebral hemispheres. *In* A. Carmazza and E. Zurif (eds.). *The Acquisition and Breakdown of Language Parallels and Divergences.* Johns Hopkins Press, Baltimore. In press.

Murrill, R. I., and Wallace, D. T. 1971. A method of making an endocranial cast through the foramen magnum of an intact skull. *Am. J. Phys. Anthropol. 34:*441–446.

Oyen, O. J., and Walker, A. 1977. Stereometric craniometry. *Am. J. Phys. Anthropol. 46:*177–182.

Radinsky, L. 1968. Evolution of somatic sensory specialization in otter brains. *J. Comp. Neurol. 134:*495–506.

Radinsky, L. 1970. The fossil evidence of prosimian brain evolution. *In* C. R. Noback, and W. Montagna (eds.). *The Primate Brain.* Appleton-Century-Croft, New York. Pp. 209–224.

Radinsky, L. 1971. An example of parallelism in carnivore brain evolution. *Evolution 25,* 518–522.

Radinsky, L. 1972. Endocasts and studies of primate brain evolution. *In* R. H. Tuttle (ed.). *Functional and Evolutionary Biology of Primates.* Alding-Atherton, Chicago. Pp. 175–184.

Radinsky, L. 1974a. Prosimian brain morphology: Functional and phylogenetic implications. *In* R. D. Martin, G. A. Doyle, and A. C. Walker (eds.). *Prosimian Biology.* Duckworth, London. Pp. 781–798.

Radinsky, L. 1974b. The fossil evidence of anthropoid brain evolution. *Am. J. Phys. Anthropol. 41:*15–28.

Radinsky, L. 1975a. Evolution of the felid brain. *Brain Behav. Evol. 11:*214–254.

Radinsky, L. 1975b. Viverrid neuroanatomy: Phylogenetic and behavioral implications. *J. Mammal. 56:*130–150.

Radinsky, L. 1975c. Primate brain evolution. *Am. Sci. 63:*656–663.

Radinsky, L. 1977. Early primate brains: Facts and fiction. *J. Hum. Evol. 6:*79–86.

Saban, R. 1976. A Propos des Traces Vasculaires Endocraniennes chez l'Homme de Rabat. IX Congres USIPP, Nice, Coll. 6. Les Plus Anciens Hominides. Pretirage. Pp. 430–444.

Saban, R. 1977. The place of Rabat man (Kebibat, Morocco) in human evolution. *Curr. Anthropol. 18*(3):518–524.

Sacher, G. 1970. Allometric and factorial analysis of brain structure in insectivores and primates. *In* C. R. Noback, and W. Montagna (eds.). *The Primate Brain.* Appleton-Century-Crofts, New York. Pp. 245–287.

Schepers, G. W. H. 1946. Part II in the *South African Fossil Ape-Man* by R. Broom. *Transvaal Mus. Mem. 2.*

Schepers, G. W. H. 1950. Part II in Broom, R. Robinson, J. T. and Schepers, G. W. H. *Sterkfontein Ape-man Pleisianthropus. Transvaal Mus. Mem. 4.*

Schepers, G. W. H. 1952. Part II. *The braincasts in ape-man of Swartkrans. Transvaal Mus. Mem. 6.*

Shellshear, V. L., and Smith, G. E. 1934. A comparative study of the endocranial cast of Sinanthropus. *Philos. Trans. R. Soc. London Ser. B 223:*469.

Teszer, D., Tzauaras, A., Gruner, J., and Hecaen, H. 1972. L'asymétrie droite–gauche du planum temporale. A propos de l'étude anatomique de 100 cerveaux. *Rev. Neurol. 126:*444–449.

von Bonin, G. 1963. *The Evolution of the Human Brain.* University of Chicago Press, Chicago.

Tobias, P. V. 1971. *The Brain in Hominid Evolution.* Columbia University Press, New York.

Welker, W. I., and Campos, G. B. 1963. Physiological significance of sulci in somatic sensory cerebral cortex in mammals of the family Procyonidae. *J. Comp. Neurol. 120:*19–36.

Yeni-Komshian, G. H., and Benson, D. A. 1976. Anatomical study of cerebral asymmetry in the temporal lobe of humans, chimpanzees, and rhesus monkeys. *Science 192:*387–389.

Index

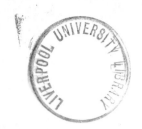